# The Complete Guide to Fall Prevention™

### "Everything You Need To Know To Remain Independent"

# 3-part Guide designed to Reduce Fall Risk and Improve Balance & Stability

By
Kelly Ward, M.S., Therapeutic Aging
The Fall Prevention Lady

*The Complete Guide to Fall Prevention*™

Copyright © 2012 by Kelly Ward

Published by:

> Kelly Ward
> P.O. Box 191655
> Sacramento, CA 95819
> Info@TheFallPreventionLady.com
> www.TheFallpreventionLady.com

First Printing, 2012

Printed in the United State of America

ISBN: 0985602511                    (10 digit)
      978-0-9856025-1-2             (13 digit)

Cover Design by Leslie Sears
General Editing by Mike Rounds

# Contents

# Dedication

They say it takes a village to raise a child; well it took a community to produce this book! I couldn't have written this without the help of my class participants and in-home training clients. Their struggles and achievements while balance training inspired me to share the process with others.

Thank you all for the opportunity to work with and learn from you. And thank you for posing for the pictures! You all passed your mid-term exam!

In all things, I give glory to Jesus Christ, my savoir, my source, my strength. Thank you for my passion, my purpose, and my fall prevention vision. My hope is in the Lord.

This Complete Guide to Fall Prevention™ is also dedicated to some people who have made a significant difference in my life. I dedicate this book to my father, Brigadier General Jerry E. Ward, who is also in heaven guiding my steps.

A special thanks to my mother, Jean Allred, for listening to my frustrations and fears and believing in my vision.

Thank you to my step-mother, Carol Anderson-Ward, for encouraging me to stick with my dreams when I felt like giving up.

Coach White, my high school basketball coach, thanks for teaching me to hang in there and never give up.

Mostly, thanks to Dr. Debra Rose, the creator of the FallProof™. This program has blessed my life.

Thanks also to my fitness mentors, Paul Chek, Gary Gray, Rodney Corn, and Craig Ballantyne. Your training techniques have shaped my training philosophy.

## About the Author

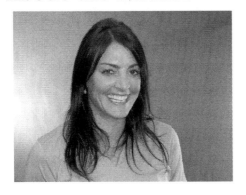

Introducing Kelly Ward, The Fall Prevention Lady™, who is a national public speaker, health educator and fall prevention consultant.

She is a Health Educator with a Bachelor of Science degree in Public Health, from West Chester University, PA and a Master of Science degree in Therapeutic Aging from California State University, Sacramento; a program that combines Gerontology and Therapeutic Recreation to promote healthy aging through lifestyle modifications.

She has appeared on cable television shows as a balance & mobility specialist and teaches small group balance and mobility training classes in the Sacramento area. She provides in-home specialized instruction and fall prevention training to older adults, training for trainers and continuing education programs for staff members.

She's a certified Fallproof™ Balance and Mobility specialist. *(You can read more about Fallproof™ in the Resource Section)* She's a Certified Therapeutic Recreation Specialist (CTRS) and gerontologist specializing in the aging process and developing programs for that meet the needs facing older adults.

She's a Certified Personal Fitness trainer with certifications from AFAA (Aerobic and Fitness Association of America) and the Senior Fitness Association.

More importantly, she's the Fall Prevention Lady™ who is passionate about educating seniors and facilitating a fall prevention lifestyle. In other words, she's really busy and probably more concerned about preventing you from falling down than you are.

Impressed? Yes? No? Maybe? Don't care?

Well, let's stop talking about Kelly and start talking about falls and how to prevent them.

## About the Book

***The Complete Guide to Fall Prevention*™** is for anyone who has fallen or who is concerned about falling, regardless of age or physical condition.

I wrote this book to be educational, entertaining, and easy to read. I've done my best to make the exercises, and their benefits for you, easy to understand and the resources useful for you to use in your life.

My hope is that after reading the guide you will find preventing falls easy to do.

More importantly, I hope it helps to keep you from falling and injuring yourself!

You may be reading this guide for your own safety or because you are concerned about your spouse, a parent, a grandparent, an uncle or an aunt, or an elderly neighbor.

Whatever your reason for reading, I want to congratulate you for wanting to learn more about how to keep yourself and loved ones free from falls and independent within the home.

Comedians make jokes about falling and there may be a lot of funny stories about falling but regardless of how much you laugh at them, **falls are serious!**

---

- 1 in 3 adults over the age of 65 living at home will fall each year
- 2 out of 3 residents in assisted living facilities falls each year
- 1 of 2 people over 80 will fall each year

**That's a LOT of falls!**

---

Although falls are associated with the aging process, **they are not a normal or necessary part of growing old!**

There is usually an underlying cause or external hazard that increases the possibility of losing your balance.

These causes and threats are referred to as fall risk factors and the more risk factors you have, the greater the chance of falling

**The good news is that up to 55% of falls can be prevented**

Educating yourself about falls and fall risk factors is the first and most important step you can take to remain independent.

## WHO'S FALLING?

First let me explain that ***not all old people are the same***. Aging is a unique process for everyone and we have:

- Different values
- Different genetics
- Different lifestyles
- Different medical conditions
- Different coping mechanisms
- Been through different circumstances
- Made different daily choices

There are different cohorts of "old people" with different values. A value is something that a person regards as important and these values shape a person's behavior.

For example, many older adults do not value exercise because they haven't recognized the benefits, either short or long term.

*Here's a gold star tip: Consistent exercise is the #1 way to reduce the risk of a fall and remain independent!*

As an adult child, you may find it extremely difficult to get mom or dad to participate in an activity program because they **do not:**

- Value the behavior
- Believe they can do the behavior
- Believe they will benefit from the behavior
- Think it's right for adults to be taking orders from their kids or younger caregivers because no matter how old we get, they're still the younger generation

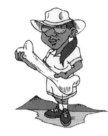
And men, don't think this is just for women! In days of old, it wasn't socially acceptable for a woman to sweat and to work hard.

But thanks to the women's revolution,

### STRONG IS THE NEW SKINNY!

If you value your independence, I hope that this book encourages you to make some lifestyle changes.

While I have your attention, let me briefly explain the different age demographics because some of these differences may affect how everyone gets along:

### Young-old:

- The young-old are anywhere between 50-74 years old
- They are the "baby boomers" who used to be "hippies"
- They are more educated about the benefits of exercise

- Yet, despite their knowledge about the health benefits of a consistent exercise program, **less than 25% of baby boomers get the recommended amounts of daily activity**

### Consider this...

The **choices you make** or how you live your life during one decade (your 60s) will **determine your VITALITY** in the following decade (your 70s).

For boomers, choosing to be active during these years can *directly impact the quality of life* after retirement.

### Old:

- The "old" are categorized as being between 75-84 years of age
- They are the Silent Generation; the parents of boomers
- This is a time when **dignity is struggling to be preserved**
- This group has heard about the benefits of exercise but may not know how to exercise safely or correctly...if at all!

At an age when being active or not can determine one's level of independence, it was reported that over **15% of this group gets no physical activity while only 20% report some physical activity.**

Once you decide to get active, **the benefits of exercise include:**

- More energy and improved moods
- Better management of chronic diseases
- Improved digestion and elimination
- Improved sleep patterns
- Fewer or no falls
- The ability to REMAIN INDEPENDENT

## Old-old:

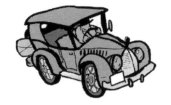

- Is anyone over the age of 85
- ***Demographically, this is fastest growing segment of the population***
- They are the GI Generation who grew up before TV, lived through two World Wars, the Great Depression, Vietnam, plus every societal change and major invention that has occurred in the past century
- Resilient is the most common adjective used to describe this group
- Even though this group benefits the MOST from physical activity and strengthening programs, 30% of this group gets NO physical activity and only 10% report some activity

That means that **60% of the fastest growing segment of the population gets zero to minimal amounts of exercise, movement or activity.**

### *Hey! Guess what? It's never too late to start!*

Sure, changes occur and there may have been some debilitating circumstances but modifications can be made!
You can still do something!

### *Make movement part of your daily routine.*

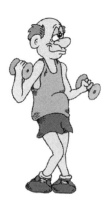

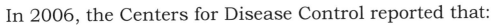

## PART I: EDUCATION ABOUT FALLING

### The Facts About Falls

Did you know:
- Every 15 seconds, a senior is treated in the emergency room due to a fall?
- Every 35 minutes, an older adult dies as a result of a fall?

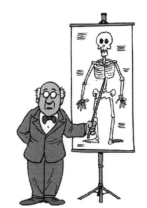

In 2006, the Centers for Disease Control reported that:
- More than one third of adults over 65 who live at home will fall at least once per year
- 24% of people who fall report a serious injury and require hospitalization

Falls are:
- The leading cause of injury death among adults over 65
- The most common cause of non–fatal injuries and hospital admissions for trauma

Falls injure people so badly that 40% of people who fall will not be able to live independently again and 70% will require assistance in activities of daily living after a fall.

As a result, many falls result in the premature institutionalization due to:
- Loss of independence
- Reduced quality of life due to the fear of falling again.

### Falls are quickly becoming a PUBLIC HEALTH EPIDEMIC!

By 2025, it is estimated that one in five Americans will be over 65 years old and the population over the age of 85 doubles every 30 years.

As the number of aging baby boomers increases, the need for programs that encourage individuals to make lifestyle changes to reduce the risk of accidental falls is undeniable.

## The Cost Of Falls

While an accidental fall can cost a person their independence, non-fatal fall services such as emergency response care, hospital-related medical services, and physician care cost society billions of dollars and the burden of these costs is passed onto taxpayers.

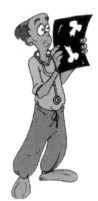

In 2000, direct medical costs of falls totaled over $19 billion:

- $179 million for fatal falls
- $19 billion for nonfatal fall injuries

In 2001, Medicare paid over $4.7 billion for fall related hip fractures and it's estimated that cost will reach $32.4 billion in 2020 and as much as $240 billion in 2040.

Fall-related hospital admission rates increase with age.

- In 2000, 39% of older adults who were admitted to a hospital after a fall were over 85 years of age
- 20% of older Californians die within one year after a hip fracture
- 25% of people who break their hip are still in a nursing home one year later
- In 2008, the average annual rate for a private nursing home room was $76,460
- The cost to live in a skilled nursing home is increasing approximately four percent per year!

Ironically, **over 50% of these falls might have been prevented** by:
- Learning about fall risk factors
- Beginning a fall prevention exercise program

# Planning For An Accident?

You probably aren't planning for an accident but remember, all falls are accidents (unless you're a movie stuntman) so the best thing you can do is plan ahead in case of an accident.

I have a 90-year old client who fell and broke her hip.  While in the hospital, she caught pneumonia and while in rehab, caught a highly infectious strain of diarrhea and was ultimately removed from her home for nearly six weeks.

Thankfully, she had planned ahead. As a result, her long distance relatives knew exactly what needed to be done at the house so she could focus her energies on recovery.

## The Advanced Care Directive (ACD)

The importance of having an Advanced Care Directive cannot be over emphasized.  An Advanced Care Directive is a legal document prepared by an adult in case of a medical crisis, before any crisis has occurred.

The ACD is a detailed outline of the adult's wishes and how things are to be carried out if they are incompetent or unable to make decisions.

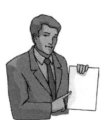

The ACD precisely defines:
- Do not resuscitate orders
- Life prolonging measures in case of coma
- Organ donations
- Who makes medical decisions for the person
- Estate concerns
- 

The power of stating your wishes cannot be ignored. Believe it or not but people cannot read your mind!  Loved ones don't know what you want or how you want something handled unless they are told.

**There is nothing worse than suddenly being removed from your world and placed in a cold, sterile environment where you don't know what will happen next.**

When a person ends up in the hospital or rehab hospital, this is when they need *positive thoughts* and *words of encouragement* more than ever.

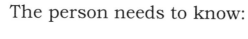

The person needs to know:

- **The fall wasn't their fault**
- Everything will be ok
- **They can and will recover**
- Everything will be ok
- **They're lucky to be alive**
- Everything will be OK

Regardless of the injury, the person who fell will replay the fall incident over and over in their mind, wishing they would have done something differently.

For those who are lucky to be released within a few hours or days, the fear of falling again can be as paralyzing as a serious injury. See page 33 for more about the psychological fear of falling.

## Advanced Planning:

While no one plans on falling, accidents happen. Similar to other emergencies, a person should plan ahead in case they are not able to return home after a fall, especially if they live alone.

If a person has no nearby relatives, they might want to talk to a neighbor or a trustworthy friend about some situations in case of an accident.

Here is a checklist of things that an older adult who lives alone may want to arrange for in case of a fall.

Have someone ready to:

1. Let the animals outside and inside
2. Water the plants
3. Pay the bills (mortgage first)
4. Check thermostat
5. Pick up mail
6. Remember to leave them the contact information for:
   1. Family and friends that need to be notified
   2. The name and number of a veterinarian
   3. The name and number of a preferred kennel name and location in case of a long term absence

**Mostly, invest in a medical alert system such as Lifeline or Vital-Link in case of a fall!**

With some advanced planning, anyone who falls can rest easier and concentrate all their energy on recovery because things at home are under control.

## Planning For Future Falls:

Every fall is different and every person who falls is different.
Just as there are numerous causes for a fall, there are numerous
ways to reduce the risk of an accidental fall.

Fall prevention researchers have determined that addressing two or
more fall risk factors significantly reduces the risk of losing your
balance. You do this by implementing two or more of the following:

- Education about falls and fall risk factors
- Modifying the home environment
- Managing medications
- Participating in a fall prevention exercise routine

## REMEMBER, it's estimated that over 50% of falls can be prevented!

## THINGS THAT CAUSE FALLS

Extensive research has determined that there are two types of fall risk factors:

1. External, (or Extrinsic) causes
2. Internal, (or Intrinsic) factors

Some factors you can change and some you cannot.

> **God, grant me the wisdom to accept the things I cannot change,**
>
> **the courage to change the things I can, and**
>
> **the wisdom to know the difference.**

### External Causes For Falls

External causes for falls are
- Outside of the individual
- Situations a person usually has some type of control over

### The Home Environment

There's no place like home, there's no place like home! We love our homes.

In fact, **80%** of older adults want to remain in their homes until death. One of the most popular concepts in the aging industry is "aging in place" because this gives people what they want; people want to grow old and die in the comforts of home.

Even though senior living communities have improved tremendously in the past decade, I don't know many older adults who want to voluntarily move into an assisted living facility.

Unfortunately, there may come a time when moving into a more assisted environment is necessary (like after a fall) but for the most part, most older adults want to remain in their homes as long as possible.

With that said, the importance of creating a safe environment cannot be understated.

It is estimated that approximately 60% of falls occur in the home and the most common environmental issues are surface and lighting-related.

These are the **HIGH FALL RISK FACTORS:**
- Dim lighting
- Slippery floors
- Obstacles in the pathway

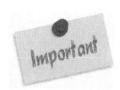

Throw Rugs

One of the best fall prevention tips is to pick up throw rugs. While these decorative ornaments can enhance the beauty of your home, these little mats can also be a safety hazard.

As we get older, we tend to drag our toes, not picking up our feet when stepping onto a new surface, especially in the comfort of our home.

We get lazy walking around the house so even though you know the throw rug is in the hallway between the kitchen and the dining room (it's been there for 15 years), you may not be paying attention or you may be tired and your toe might get caught on the end of your favorite family throw rug and cause you to fall.

You have two choices:
- You can get rid of the throw rug
- You can buy double-sided adhesive tape and secure the rug to the floor

Now comes the tough part, you have to decide.

Night Lights

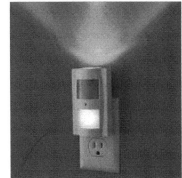

Another common fall prevention tip is to use nightlights. These glow lights plug into any outlet and can save your life in the middle of night because they illuminate your pathway.

Even though you may have lived in the same house for over 30 years and know every square inch of the journey from your bed to the bathroom, using a nightlight just makes sense. And it keeps you safe!

It's happened to all of us....you wake up in the middle of the night and you have to go to the bathroom. Urgently! You're in a hurry, your eyes haven't adjusted to the darkness and you are still half asleep.

If something was accidentally left in the pathway or a beloved pet is asleep on the floor, the chances of falling are huge if these obstacles cannot be seen.

A nightlight illuminates pathways so that trip hazards can be seen and avoided. Nightlights can be purchased at hardware and home improvement stores and many senior agencies give them out at health fairs and as promotional tools.

Bathroom

What room do you think most falls occur? If you answered, the bathroom, you are correct! (And you're welcome for the huge hint with the subtitle!)

Stepping into and out of the shower or bathtub can be frightful experiences. Cramped spaces can make movement difficult and low toilet seats can be a nightmare. Luckily, there are simple home modifications that can make the bathroom safe again.

Bathroom Modifications:

1.  *Grab bars* - These provide handholds to help with standing, sitting, or getting up. You can install them yourself or by a private contractor or non-profit agencies such as Rebuilding Together.

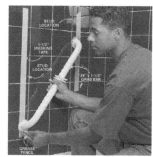

2.  *Toilet risers* - Because leg strength diminishes with age, sitting down and getting up to take care of business can be difficult, if not scary.

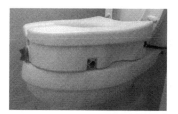

These 4-6 inch gadgets attach to the existing toilet seat and don't require professional installation. The good news is that you don't have to buy a new toilet to feel safe again
Toilet risers can be removed if you are expecting company and easy removal makes cleaning easy.

3.  *Walk-in Tubs* - Although this bathroom modification isn't cheap, a walk-in tub can make taking a bath a pleasure once again and for some, the feeling of a hot bat is invaluable! There are reputable distributors who offer professional installation in as little as 6 hours.

4.  *Floor to Ceiling bars*– If the **problem** is that you can't get out of your bed or favorite recliner without help, the **solution** is to have a floor-to-ceiling pole installed so you can grab the pole with your arms and use your upper body strength to pull yourself up without help. Most manufacturers provide professional installation.

*Important*

**People want to age with dignity.
Getting older can be difficult to accept.
Asking for help isn't always easy.**

## Entrance Steps

If you cannot feel the ground under your feet, you have no way of knowing if your foot is entirely on the step unless you look down.

Poor vision or wearing bi-focals can make it difficult to see where one step ends and one begins and a busy carpet pattern can enhance this problem.

The remedy is to put bright, and I mean **BRIGHT** neon tape on the edges of the stairs so you can clearly see where EACH step ends.

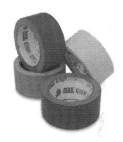

This modification is easy and cheap and can save your life if you have peripheral neuropathy, loss of feeling or painful sensations in your feet.

When you can no longer use steps safely, a ramp can be installed. These require professional installation and can be quite costly however some non-profit agencies can install these for free or at a reduced cost.   (See the Resource section)

Making modifications to your home and using assistive living tools are not signs of weakness, but tools to independence.

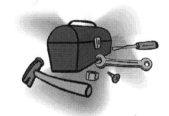

It can be humbling to recognize you are not as strong as you once were and it takes courage to ask for help....

### REMEMBER THAT HELP IS AVAILABLE!

---

### BONUS REPORT:  Home Safety Checklist

Go through the Home Safety Checklist in the INDEX and make the recommended changes.

It's up to you.  Have courage.

---

## Shoes and Footwear

The shoes you wear can increase your risk of a fall. Your shoes are like tires for your car; they need to be changed routinely.

If you are still wearing the sneakers you bought in 2005 or got for Christmas two years ago, it's time for a new pair!

Your feet change and grow (and shrink) so it's important that you have a good fit.

---

### REAL LIFE

I have a dedicated client who is very pro-active in her fall prevention efforts.

She knows the severity of a fall because while rushing into church she fell and fractured her hip. After replaying the incident, she realized she was doing too many things at once; rushing, talking, and not paying attention when she stopped to change directions.

After we talked, it became apparent that it was her NON-SKID shoes that caused her to fall when she suddenly stopped. Her foot stuck to the floor and her body kept going!

---

Recommended Fall Prevention Shoe Checklist:

- Lightweight (rubber shoes are heavier than nylon)
- Wear tie ups or Velcro-fastener (Slip-on shoes increase fall risk)
- Texturized sole to reduce slips
- Have wide heel
- Provide ankle support
- Are not too tight but allow some wiggle in your toes.
- Do not cause friction on heel when walking (too big)
- Do not have high heels or extra thick soles
- Do not have super soft or slippery soles (worn out shoes are slick, especially on wet surface)

- How NON-SKID is the bottom of your shoe?
- What type of activity will you be wearing it for?
- Where you will wear the shoe?

While good arch support is important, I like shoes that are flexible.

A "flexible" shoe has some bend when you grab the toe and the heel and try to bend the shoe in half.

There are conflicting recommendations for proper footwear and as a personal fitness trainer, I may suggest something that might seem strange because it's different than what you're used to or it's a relatively new research-based finding.

The final decision is up to you but I want to tell you about some new footwear and how to maximize your safety while getting the most out of your training efforts.

I wear **Nike Free Sneakers™ or Vibram 5-fingers™** for training because the sole is extremely flexible which works the deep inner muscles of my calves and feet.

**Please note: Barefoot training and wearing Nike Free sneakers are not appropriate for everyone.**

I do not have any foot problems or structural issues so I really like barefoot training when I do my balance training because:
- I can feel the ground under my feet
- It really works my calf muscles
- It builds my ankle strength

If you see a podiatrist, please talk with talk with him/her about proper fitting shoes and your footwear options.

People living with diabetes and those with permanent nerve damage in their lower extremities need to take extra pre-cautions with their feet.

**If you wear doctor-prescribed inserts, use them!**

A WARNING ABOUT INSERTS!

If you experience knee and/or hip pain shortly after wearing inserts, talk to your doctor.

Inflexible ankles and stiff calf muscles that don't move correctly cause the body to compensate or make adjustments. This stiffness and inflexibility affects how you move and put you at an increased risk of a fall.

Prolonged compensation results in inefficient movement patterns that start with your foot and are passed up to your knee, then to your hip and even to your shoulder.

So if your hip or shoulder starts to hurt after you begin wearing a pair of shoe inserts, please talk to your doctor!!!

## Nutrition

*"Food to your body is like gasoline to your car; the higher quality of gasoline, the better the engine runs"* ~ K.Ward

We know what we're supposed to eat and we've been hearing it for years.

Our parents told us, our grandparents told us, the media reminds us and our doctors prescribe it for us.

Remember the food pyramid? Although the structure of the pyramid has changed in recent years, the message is the same.

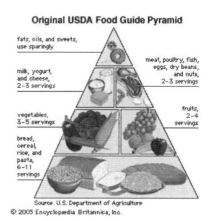

The better your diet, the better you will feel and function.

I'm not a dietician but I am knowledgeable about nutrition from my collegiate studies, personal fitness training, holistic lifestyle studies and personal experiences.

I'm not going to tell you anything new but I am going to recommend that you try to adhere to these guidelines:

- Eat fresh vegetables and fruits
- Eat lean proteins such as fish, chicken, turkey, beans, egg whites (yolks are ok now, too)
- Eat high fiber foods
- Low fat foods
- Minimize sugars, artificial sweeteners and transfats in diet
- Stay away from products with high fructose corn syrup (soda, candy, baked goods)

Since this book is about fall prevention, be sure to include bone-building food sources that are high in calcium, especially if you have osteoporosis (weak, thin, fragile bones).

Foods high in calcium include:

- Dairy products
- Sardines
- Broccoli
- Cod liver oil
- Calcium-fortified cereals and juices

As a holistic lifestyle coach, I recommend that you **avoid eating processed foods.**

In the past 10 years, there have been over 1,000 new food additives invented. Our body doesn't recognize these chemicals and cannot digest them.

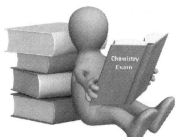

A good rule of thumb is to look at the ingredients and if you cannot pronounce the first five or need to use a chemistry book to read the ingredients, the food is highly processed.

Also, the longer the shelf life, the worse the food is for your body.

You don't have to break the bank to eat healthy. If possible, grow a garden or shop for fruits and vegetables at local farmers markets.

When preparing meals, try to steam, bake or sauté rather than fry. Go easy on the sauces and condiments and try to stay away from fast food meals and all soda and colas.

## MODERATION IS THE KEY

Water

*"Just as food to the body is like gasoline to the car, water to the body is like oil to the car engine!!!"*~ K.Ward

- The brain is up to 85% water
- Muscles are up to 70% water

Vital processes in the body that require water include digestion, respiration, circulation and elimination

As we age, our thirst mechanism doesn't work as efficiently and we don't realize we are thirsty until it's too late. If you're feeling lethargic or not thinking clearly, it could be because you are partially dehydrated!

It is recommended that adults drink **half of their bodyweight in fluid ounces each day**, more if you are physically active or the weather is hot and humid.  For example, if a person weighs 140 pounds.  How many fluid ounces should she drink every day?

---

### TOO MUCH VS. NOT ENOUGH

Please note that there are some medical conditions that do not encourage excessive fluid intake.

- Congestive heart failure is one such condition
- If you are on diuretics, talk to your doctor about fluid intake levels.

### BUT I'M INCONTINENT....

Unfortunately, loss of bladder control is an issue some of us have to deal with as we age.  It's not only embarrassing but also causes pre-mature institutionalization.

- You may try to limit fluid intake in hopes this will reduce urine output.
- Restricting fluids may seem logical but can be dangerous to the urinary tract if the fluids are not replaced.
- The more concentrated your urine (due to dehydration) the more irritating that can be to your urinary tract.

### Remember, the body needs water to function!

(Answer: 70)

## Pets

You are probably not going to want to hear this. In fact, you will probably skip right over this section but I have to mention it because your beloved pet could be a major fall risk.

Pets are like family and they miss you when you're gone.

They show their adoration the second you walk into the door; dogs jump up and down and cats rub against you because they just want to touch you!

Unfortunately, they can get wrapped up in your legs and cause you to trip.

- Your cat might stop in your pathway when you are walking
- The dog might take a nap in an unlikely place and cause you to stumble.
- The cat might rub against the legs of your walker and lay down between the wheels.
- You might not hear the dog running up behind you, turn directly into him and fall down.

## BY NO MEANS AM I TELLING YOU TO GET RID OF YOUR BELOVED FAMILY PET.

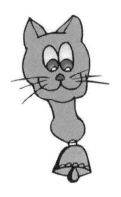

I AM suggesting that you put a bell on the pet's collar so you hear him coming.

If you have fallen more than twice because of your pet, you have to ask yourself if that pet is worth your well-being, safety and independence or even your life.

The choice is yours.

## Activity Level

Living an active lifestyle is recommended for people of all ages but is especially important for older adults.

Due to the physical decline associated with the aging process, you must make a conscious decision to make exercise part of your daily routine if you want to stay independent.

The benefits of being in an exercise program include:

- Increased energy levels
- Manage chronic disease
- Reduce risk of falls
- Group support

To prevent falls, there are four (4) kinds of exercise you must do:

- Flexibility or range of motion training
- Strength or resistance training
- Balance training
- Endurance training

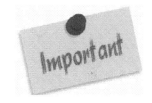

Plus, practice posture awareness!

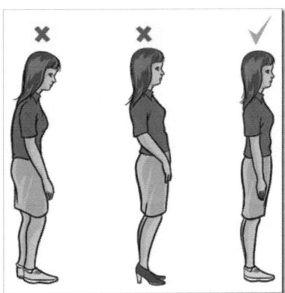

## Internal Or Intrinsic Fall Risk Factors

These are processes going on within the individual. Some intrinsic fall risk factors cannot be changed but can be managed.

### Attitude

You control your attitude. You can decide if you will be positive or negative-minded, if you will be happy or sad. Your thoughts influence your behavior. If you think you can do a task and believe in yourself, you are more likely to be able to complete the task.

The power of your thoughts cannot be understated. It's kind of like the book, "The Secret"; if you think positive thoughts, you bring positive things into your life.

If you *see yourself as independent and able,* you are more likely to become that.
If you think you're going to fall, if you constantly think about falling, if you envision yourself falling, you will probably fall.

### "I CANT'S"....

As a balance and mobility specialist, I work with some people who have a serious case of the **"I cants".** I observe this condition when I ask class participants or training clients to do a challenging activity. I'll hear:

- "**I can't** do this and close my eyes"
- "**I can't** stand without holding onto the chair"
- "**I can't** walk without my walker"
- "**I can't** stand up without using my hands"

If you convince yourself that you can't do something, it is highly likely that you will not be able to do it until you are pushed out of your comfort zone and you prove yourself wrong.

The Cycle of Fear

When a person falls, they become terrified of falling again so they limit activities that might cause them to fall. The less activity a person gets, the weaker they become. Restricted activity leads to isolation.

Missing social interaction can lead to depression and depressed people are at greater risk of falling.

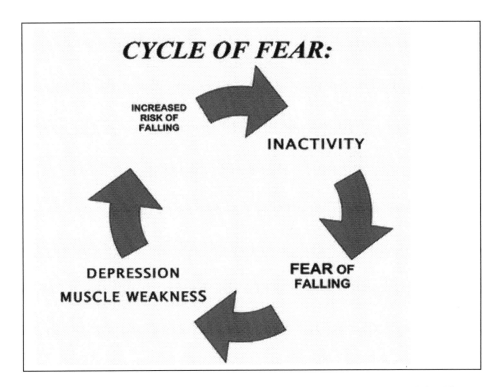

You have some control over your fears but the fear of falling can be difficult to conquer. If your fear of falling interferes with your activities of daily living, it's time to get help.

For the person who can't just "get over it", there's help! "Matter of Balance™" is a nationally acclaimed program that addresses the psychological fears associated with falling.

For more about "Matter of Balance™" see the Resource section.

**THIS IS A VICIOUS CYCLE THAT MUST BE BROKEN**

## Overconfidence

At the other end of the spectrum is overconfidence.

Some older adults don't think they'll fall because that's what happens to "old people" and some of these people are in their 70s, 80s and even 90s.

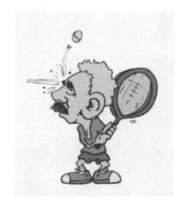

These are prior athletes or those currently engaging in regular activity programs who may not fully realize their physical limitations.

Sometimes a person is in denial about getting old and does not realize (cannot accept) that the body doesn't function or react like it did years ago.

Ultimately these individuals put themselves in risky situations.

While there is no program to deal with this overconfidence, an increased awareness of **actual physical condition** can be an eye opener for some.

I use the Senior Fitness Tests to assess current fitness levels.

These standardized tests are designed specifically for older adults and show how a person is aging in comparison to people of similar age and gender. See page 51 for more information on testing.

Try taking a few to see how you do!

**Check your attitude and don't let
the fear of falling or overconfidence increase the risk of
a fall!**

## State of Mind (Your Brain and Mental Process)

Unfortunately, our body isn't the only thing that slows down with age. There are age-related changes that occur in our brain and thought processes, too.

Some common cognitive impairments associated with the aging process are:

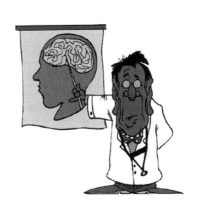

- Inability to recall appropriate responses quickly
- Difficulty dividing attention between two or more tasks
- Impaired ability to "think on the fly" or solve problems on the move.

These age-related cognitive delays also affect the ability to anticipate and react appropriately if you are accidentally pushed at the mall, bumped into while grocery shopping or come to a sudden stop when using public transportation.

Multi Tasking Concerns

Fall prevention research demonstrates that we lose the ability to divide attention between different tasks and our balance as we age.

In other words, you pay more attention to what you're doing (carrying groceries) rather than maintaining balance.

The good news is that following a consistent balance training program can improve your mind-to-muscle response and reduce the risk of a fall.

Like other motor skills, balance can improve with practice.

Real Life

Falling down is not your first concern when you are
unloading groceries, talking on the phone and
calling the dog.

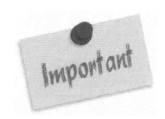

If you're tired, you might not pick up your toes and
trip over the curb or you may not see the dog as
you're walking into the house.

The result can be a life-changing fall!

## Presence of Medical Conditions

Chronic diseases can be hereditary or the result of accumulated
lifestyle choices.   The risk of living with a chronic disease increases
with age because the body is more vulnerable and takes longer to
recover due to weakened immune systems.

Living with multiple medical conditions is an intrinsic
fall risk factor because disease stresses the body's
internal environment.

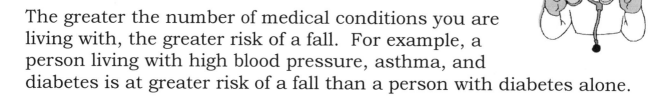

The greater the number of medical conditions you are
living with, the greater risk of a fall.  For example, a
person living with high blood pressure, asthma, and
diabetes is at greater risk of a fall than a person with diabetes alone.

The reason is that the first person's body is under more stress and
can be weakened as a result.

## Medication Management

Doctors prescribe medications to slow the progression of the disease
process and to manage chronic disease symptoms.

Obviously the more conditions a person is living with, the greater
number of medications s/he is probably taking. The more
medications a person is taking, the greater the risk of side effects.

## Taking four (4) or more medications daily is an intrinsic fall risk factor

You need the medications but the main side effects are:
- Dizziness
- Light-headedness
- Drowsiness

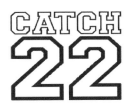

Obviously, these side effects increase the risk of a fall. You need the medication but you don't want to fall.

Thus, managing your medications is vital to your safety and independence.

### Remember: Management begins with education!

### Option #1: Educate yourself about:

- <u>Proper dosage</u>. Due to slowed drug clearance times (kidney function) in the older body, an adult dose is half of the recommended amount (over the counter). Check with your doctor about dosage amounts & review medications regularly
- <u>Timing of medication.</u> Make sure you are taking each medication at the correct time of the day
- <u>Food-drug interactions</u>. Some foods interfere with the metabolism of some drugs
- <u>Primary organ</u> that is affected by the drug

Be aware of the effect that each pill has on your body.

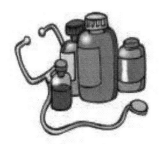

For instance, if you get dizzy when you take your blood pressure medication, you don't want to clean the house after taking it. If your heart disease medication makes you tired, you don't want to go for a walk after taking it.

## Option #2: Brown bag it!

Healthcare professionals recommend a "brown bag" day.

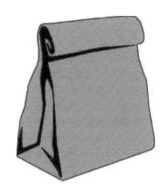

A brown bag day is when you put all your medications in a bag and go to the doctor or pharmacist.

The purpose of this is to:

- Answer any questions you have about your medications
- Check expiration dates
- See if any medications cancel out or increase the effects of each other

Check with your local senior center or Area Agency on Aging about brown day opportunities in your community.

> ***For more information, look in the index for the bonus report,***
> ***"Medications that Increase Fall Risk"***

## Advanced Age

As much as we try to fight it, there are natural declines associated with growing older.

The body isn't as flexible as it used to be, we can't run as fast let alone walk as steady.

Sometimes walking half a block can feel like the 10th mile and if a policeman asked you to walk the straight line, he would probably arrest you for suspicion of being drunk; at 10 o'clock in the morning!

> **Simply put, balance control is about senses and muscles.**
>
> To maintain balance, our senses collect information from the environment and transmit this information to the brain to be processed.
>
> The <u>brain then transmits a motor response to the muscles.</u>
>
> The speed and accuracy of sensory input transmitted for central processing of musculoskeletal response determines ability to prevent a fall.

The three sensory systems that provide input relative to balance are:

1. Vision: EYES
2. Vestibular: EARS
3. Somatosensory: FEET

### *EYES (Scientifically speaking: Our vision system)*

We are a vision-dependent society when it comes to balance.

We rely heavily on visual input for information about our body position in space and the location of objects in our environment.

Age-related changes in vision that affect your balance include a **reduction** in:

- Depth perception
- Contrast sensitivity
- Visual acuity
- Peripheral vision

An estimated one in four adults over the age of 75 reports some form of visual impairment and the three leading causes of vision impairment and loss are glaucoma, macular degeneration and cataracts.

**Glaucoma:** results in loss of peripheral vision and tunnel vision. This is how a person living with glaucoma sees:

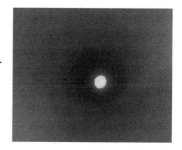

**Macular Degeneration**: results in loss of central field of vision.
There are two forms; wet and dry macular degeneration.

New surgical techniques are able to prevent total loss of vision. This is what a person living with macular degeneration sees.

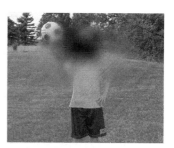

**Cataracts:** results in blurry, discolored vision. Vision is cloudy. This is how a person with cataracts views the world: (cloudy, nearsighted)

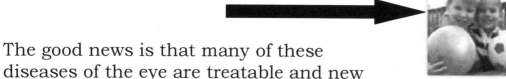
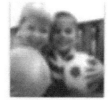

Normal Vision          Vision with Cataracts

The good news is that many of these diseases of the eye are treatable and new treatment options are increasingly available.

Early detection can greatly improve your outcome so **get regular eye exams** (at least once a year) and ask specifically to be screened for these conditions.

Since we rely mostly on visual input for balance, you MUST learn how to utilize input from the other senses while you are still able to use vision in order to reduce fall risk.

BI-FOCALS ARE A FALL RISK!

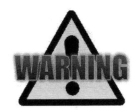

Problem: Bifocal and multifocal glasses are an increased fall risk because the near-vision lower lens segment blurs floor-level objects at critical distances thus impairing ability to detect environmental hazards.

Solution: Unifocal glasses are being used to prevent this problem so ask your ophthalmologist if you are a candidate for these lower fall risk prescription eyewear.

### EARS (Scientifically speaking: Vestibular system):

The vestibular system is located in the inner ear where there are hair cells that serve as "motion detectors".

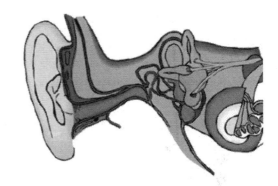

The Ear - Cut Away View

This inner ear system is activated every time you turn your head and eyes.

As we age, we lose hair cells. The result is an increased sensitivity to head movements.

If you don't experience classic vertigo dizziness symptoms, impairment in the vestibular system may go undetected until you fall.

Early detection of vestibular impairment by a physical therapist can reduce dizziness and the risk of an accidental fall.

**Please note this is a different part of the ear than the "hearing" part. You can wear hearing aids and NOT have vestibular and/or balance disorders. And you can have perfect hearing and have a vestibular impairment.**

There are new technologies available to treat vestibular disorders. You may want to check with your doctor about specific treatment options.

As a certified FallProof™ balance and mobility specialist, I teach techniques that help stabilize your gaze so it doesn't feel like you, or the world, are spinning every time you turn your head.

Being aware of the senses involved in balance is the first step to preventing accidental falls.

### FEET (Scientifically speaking: Somatosensory system):

This sensory system provides valuable information about the environment and our balance.

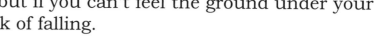

We have "position receptors" located all over the body that provide input about the body position in relation to space and these receptors are especially plentiful in the feet and the neck.

Due to age-related declines in this system, older adults have a reduced ability to feel contact between the feet and the ground.

This loss of sensation results in greater postural sway to determine body position in space.

Think about when you close your eyes...do you feel your body swaying? That is because your "position receptors" are trying to figure out where you are in space.

This sounds complicated but if you can't feel the ground under your feet, you are at greater risk of falling.

This is quickly becoming a public health concern because as the number of people living with diabetes increases, so does the risk of living with peripheral neuropathy.

The Neuropathy Association is a wonderful resource for people living with this condition. You are not alone in your frustrations, fears and pain. Visit the website, www.neuropathy.org to find a support group in your area.

The good news is that training the other sensory systems involved in balance results in an increased awareness of body position in space and safer movements.

**What's the best way to prevent a fall?**

FOLLOW A CONSISTENT EXERCISE PROGRAM!

**Fall Prevention Exercise Program**
Balance involves communication between these three senses (eyes, ears, feet) and our muscles. To prevent falls, you must do exercises that challenge the senses and exercise the muscles.

The different types of exercise to prevent falls:

1. Build strength
2. Improve flexibility
3. Maintain endurance levels and improve walking gait
4. Challenge balance
5. Increase postural awareness

## Muscle and Strength Building

Adults need lean muscle mass to perform activities of daily living and remain independent. **Sarcopenia is the natural loss of muscle mass associated with aging.** This muscle loss can be slowed down with *consistent* strength training.

Consistent means two or three times a week, each week, for years. For life, if you want to live an independent lifestyle.

<u>Use It or Lose It</u>

- o We lose muscle mass as we age.

- o We lose approximately 5% of our muscle per muscle mass per decade after the age of 30

- o Without any type of activity, we can lose up to 20% of our muscle fiber per decade after the age of 60.

## #1 RISK FACTOR FOR FALLS:  Lower body weakness
## #1 WAY TO PREVENT FALLS:  Exercise to build muscle

### *It is <u>never</u> too late to benefit from consistent movement!*

Remember, the fastest growing segment of the population (over age 85) responds the best once a consistent strength-training program is started.

In addition to the age-related deterioration of the "muscles and senses", there are physical changes that affect our flexibility and endurance.

## Flexibility

Hardly anyone I know who is over 60 is as flexible as they used to be 20 years ago!

Why?

The sciences of anatomy and physiology prove that flexibility decreases as we age:

- Tendons and muscles lose their elasticity
- The older a person gets, the more you need to stretch.

Loss of flexibility is joint specific; increased stiffness in the ankle, knee and hip joints are more obvious because of walking gait and overall mobility is affected.

These limitations increase the risk of a fall.

Stress Kills:

Stress can also contribute to poor flexibility because mental and emotional stress is manifested within the body.

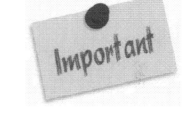

Muscles get tight, especially in the neck and shoulders, and this built up tension can result in headaches and bodyaches.

Tight muscles put increased tension on joints.

This tension results in restricted movement patterns.

**Research-based findings say the best ways to prevent falls is to minimize loss of muscle strength and joint flexibility**

### Endurance

I define endurance as the ability to do activities of daily living without fatigue or exhaustion.

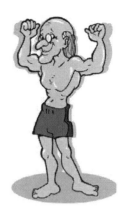

When you're tired, you are at greater risk of falling, especially when doing regular household chores.

<u>Why?</u>

Because you are less likely to pay attention to what you're doing!!!

## PAY ATTENTION TO WHAT YOU'RE DOING!

Endurance also involves your heart and lungs.

Age-related changes in heart health and lung capacity make us
- More prone to fatigue
- More prone to shortness of breath on exertion
- More susceptible to infections

The decreased capacity of the cardiovascular system results in longer recovery times after bouts of intense exercise.

It takes you longer to "bounce back" after activity. It also takes longer to recovery from injury.

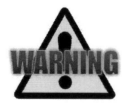

## KNOW YOUR LIMITATIONS

Walking Gait

Have you ever:

- Tripped over a rug?
- Stumbled on an uneven surface?
- Lost your balance when walking in the yard?

Walking is one of the first motor skills we learn as children and is something we take for granted as we get older, not thinking much about until a fall occurs.

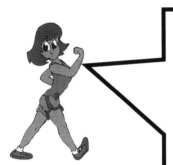

The walking gait requires leg strength to propel the body forward.

As you step from one leg to the other, balance is necessary to remain on one leg for a split second.

The foot, ankle, and calf must be strong and flexible enough to pick the foot up enough so your toes clear the floor as you step forward.

The knee must be strong and stable enough to accept your body weight as you step forward and your hip must also be flexible so one leg can stride forward as one leg remains on the ground.

Strength, flexibility, balance and endurance all affect how we walk.

- <u>Reduced leg strength</u> - You take shorter, wider steps, and begin to shuffle when you walk
- <u>Poor ankle flexibility</u> - You are unable to react to an uneven walking surface
- <u>Limited flexibility in hip, knee, and ankle</u> – You are unable to pick up your toes when you walk
- <u>Weakened hip muscles</u> - You are unsteady when you walk
- <u>Low endurance</u> - A walk around the block becomes a laborious chore rather than a leisurely stroll

Engaging in a strengthening and flexibility program, especially for the lower body, is essential to improve our walking gait.

Additionally, balance and mobility training and endurance activities are necessary in order to prevent accidental falls.

## Posture

Old age posture
We've all seen it and no one wants to have it. Shoulders rounded forward, head jutted forward and hanging toward the ground, big hump on the upper back.

If you watch this person walk, they stare at the ground and shuffle their feet.

Heck some of you reading this Guide may look like that!

The good news is that increased awareness of postural alignment can reverse that "old-age" posture as you strengthen weak postural muscles and stretch others.

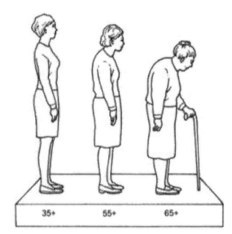

It has been demonstrated that posture affects more than the way you look. Poor posture actually puts you more off balance. Unfortunately, after years of bad postural habits, you lose the sense of true vertical because you are always starting at the floor.

I can hear you now, "but Kelly, I don't want to trip so I HAVE to look at the floor to see what's there".

No you don't!  There are training techniques that orient you to a true vertical axis and reduce your fall risk while walking.

## HAVE YOU SEEN THE MONEY FAIRY???

**A lot of people must believe in her because everyone stares at the ground or their feet while walking.**

**Stop looking!  There is no money fairy!**

In the meantime, you can practice good posture.  Good posture takes effort because it's easy to sit or stand slouched over.  Heck, everyone's doing it.  Take the road less traveled and put some effort into your posture.  You will look younger and feel better.

The benefits of proper alignment include:

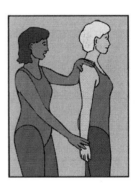

- Increased lung capacity, therefore more oxygenation to body
- Less stress and strain on your skeletal frame, joints, and muscles that hold you together
- Improved digestion due to organs being properly aligned
- Increased energy because your body doesn't have to work as hard to function

Proper posture enables you to move your body more efficiently, resulting in less fatigue thereby reducing the risk of a fall.

There are postural exercises that will help strengthen weak muscles and stretch the tight ones to correct the muscle imbalance associated with "old age" posture.

These exercises will be explained in PART 2 of this guide or you can purchase my seated stretching exercise DVD, *Take 5 for Posture*™ and follow along at home. (www.thefallpreventionlady.com)

Either way, an increased awareness of how you sit and stand throughout the day can reduce your risk of falling and **you'll look 10 years younger!**

Preventing falls requires much more than picking up throw rugs and plugging in nightlights!!!

---

**Real Life**

Dennis has Parkinson's disease. He has the typical Parkinsonism posture and is slouched forward. His chin is severely jutted forward and after years of walking like this, it is difficult for him to raise his head, lift his chin and look me in the eye (I'm six feet tall).

I'm proud to say that after only 4 of my classes with lots of verbal reminders, Dennis showed tremendous improvement. When reminded, he would sit tall, lift his chin and look forward. He walked taller and everyone in the class said he looked 10 years younger.

MJ had a stroke and her left side is paralyzed. After repeating my balance training class several times, she walked into class last week and I had to do a double take...she was standing up straight. And level! She shook her head, smiled and said, "I don't know what happened but I can stand up straight now!

---

## Summary of The Different Types of Fall Risk Factors:

### External Causes of Falls:
- Home Environment
- Shoes
- Nutrition
- Pets
- Activity Level

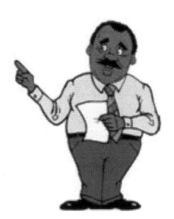

### Internal Causes of Falls:
- Attitude
- State of Mind
- Presence of Medical Conditions
- Medication Management
- Advanced Age

Unfortunately, we experience natural declines as part of getting older. The risk of permanent impairment in one or all of our balance systems increases with age.

The good news is that if one of our sensory systems is impaired, either temporarily or permanently, the efficiency of the other systems related to balance can improve with training.

Muscles can get stronger and flexibility can improve with **consistent training** and your balance skills can improve with **progressive, individualized training.**

Endurance levels increase as you faithfully follow a well-balanced exercise program.

Remember: Our bodies were made to be in motion so let's keep it that way!

Since staying active has been demonstrated to be the number one way to prevent falls, let's get started with some exercise!

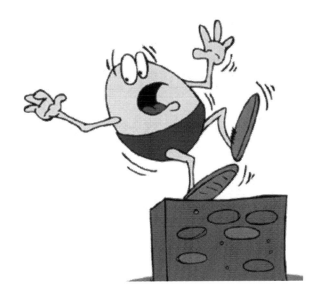

## FALL RISK SCREENING AND FITNESS ASSESSMENT

What does successful aging mean to you? To some, aging is something that just happens to them and for others, they fight it every step of the way.

### EVERYONE AGES DIFFERENTLY

Past life events and current physical abilities greatly influence the way we move and the amount of pain we feel each day. Your daily choices also affect your physical ability.

An assessment is a measure of your current physical ability. In other words, an assessment is a picture of you right now, today.

Depending on what you measure, assessment results reflect your daily choices for the past two weeks or two years!

For instance, your current weight reflects your eating habits for the past 2 weeks. That's why no one likes the scale after holiday season!

The purpose of an assessment is to gather information about you now in order to measure the effectiveness of a lifestyle or behavior change.

Assessment results provide a starting place on the journey to total body wellness and a reduced fall risk lifestyle.

The physical components of fitness related to fall risk or assessments that I suggest you measure are lower body strength and lower body flexibility.

Rome wasn't built in a day and your body didn't arrive at its current condition overnight so remember that when you test your lower body strength or lower body flexibility, the result is more reflective of your lifestyle, your daily choices, or your medical condition over the past several months or even years.

**Either way, you are who you are so be proud of it!**

I recommend using Rikli and Jones' Senior Fitness Tests to assess your physical fall risk factors because:

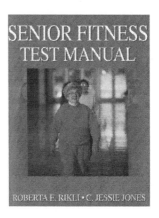

- The tests are easy to administer
- They don't require fancy equipment or a Masters degree to do them
- If the same person (you) performs the testing, test results are reliable

There are seven different Senior Fitness Tests to measure different components of functional fitness of everyday life.

Here are two quick and easy assessments that measure areas of fitness related to fall prevention.

1. **Chair Stand:** measures lower body strength. In other words, your ability to rise from chair, bed or toilet, or to catch oneself and prevent a fall.

2. **Sit and Reach:** measures lower body flexibility. In other words, your ability to perform many daily activities, your walking ability, movement speed and adjustment of balance to prevent a fall.

Test results are categorized by gender and age. This is a great way to see how you are aging in comparison to someone who is the same age and sex as you.

**For some, successful aging isn't about improving but maintaining what you have!**

If you have specific goals, these test results can motivate you to change your current fitness level.

If you are a competitive person, these test results may push you to challenge yourself.

Or, you could be like Robin and not give a hoot how you're aging in comparison to your peers or about the numbers. You just want to follow a program that will help you reduce the risk of a fall!

## HOW TO DO THE 2 ASSESSMENT TESTS

## Chair Stand

Materials: chair, stopwatch

Procedure: Sit in middle of chair, feet flat on the floor and <u>arms crossed on chest</u>. On "go", person rises to full stand then returns to fully seated position.

Do as many full stands as possible in 30 seconds. If you are more than halfway up at the end of 30 seconds, that counts as a full stand. Record number.

Adaptations: If you need to use your hands to get up, mark that in your notes.

Scoring: Write down number of chair stands done in 30 seconds and note if you used your hands.

## Sit and Reach

Materials:  Chair, 12-inch ruler

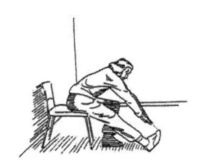

Procedure:  Sit at edge of chair.  One leg is bent with foot flat on floor and the other leg is extended straight as possible with heel on floor and toes toward ceiling.  With arms outstretched and hands overlapping, slowly bend forward reaching as far forward toward or past the toes.  Stop when knee of extended leg begins to bend.  Hold maximum reach for 2 seconds.  Practice each leg before scoring.

Scoring:  Measure distance from middle finger to top of shoe.  Midpoint at top of shoe is zero point.

If you cannot touch your toes, the number is negative.  Score is zero if you can touch your toes and the number is a positive number of inches past toes.

Take these tests, or whatever test you are able to do, record the date of testing and your results.

I sincerely hope you begin the exercise program in this *Complete Guide to Fall Prevention*™ however if you don't change a thing at all, I still want you to take the tests again in four or six weeks to see how your lifestyle is affecting your fitness, especially related to fall risk.

## Don't get discouraged; everyone has to start somewhere!

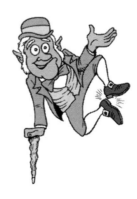

## SAFETY PRECAUTIONS

You are engaging in an **injury prevention program** so your safety is my primary concern. These guidelines are intended to keep you safe and free from injury. Please read them and take the precautions BEFORE starting the program.

### Doctor approval

Due to advanced age, the presence of medical conditions and lack of physical activity, it is important that you tell your doctor that you want to start a fall prevention exercise program.

My bet is that your doctor will be excited to hear about this since more and more doctors are writing prescriptions for the "exercise pill"

(Wishful thinking...we both know exercise doesn't come in a pill...yet!)

Once your doctor sees that these exercises are *scientifically-researched and evidence-based,* I am confident that he or she will encourage you to practice these exercises.

Doctors are busy and do not have the time to look at every exercise you are doing but I invite you to take this ***"Complete Guide To Fall Prevention™"*** to your doctor.

Please have him or her call me with any questions about the exercises or if they would like a copy of the book for the office.

Thanks in advance for spreading the word of fall prevention.

## Know Personal Limits

Your doctor said it's ok for you to begin, but realize that you know your body better than anyone! You know the difference between an *"aching pain"* and a *"something is not right pain."*

Since you know your body better than anyone, you can rate your workout at anytime and how hard you are pushing yourself. Below is the "Rate of Perceived Exertion":

| Rate of Perceived Exertion (RPE) |
| --- |
| 1   2   3   4   5   6   7   8   9   10 |
| Easy          Moderate      Too difficult |

Obviously, I don't want to you to push yourself above an 8 but when you walk with a friend, it should be difficult to carry on a conversation like you have over coffee.  Your breathing should be somewhat labored if you want to gain aerobic benefits while walking.

**Exercise does not have to be "strenuous" (RPE 6 or above) to be beneficial.**

Balance training works your central nervous system so don't expect an elevated heart rate or buckets of sweat during your workout.

Balance training can be more frustrating than anything so have patience, keep practicing and you will improve.

## Sturdy Chair

Due to the nature of the training, it is important that you create a safe environment to practice. A safe environment requires a sturdy chair or solid surface such as a countertop or hutch nearby when performing the standing exercises.

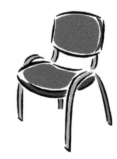

If you are unsteady on your feet or just beginning, I recommend that you practice the standing exercises between the sturdy chair and a wall when doing some of the balance exercises. The wall is there so you don't lose your balance in a backward direction.

## Proper Form

Good movement requires good form. Unfortunately our body has compensated to years of bad habits and poor posture. The result is poor movement patterns that have become automatic.

**The good news is that with increased awareness, you CAN improve the efficiency of your movements.**

## Introducing the "Form Sergeant"

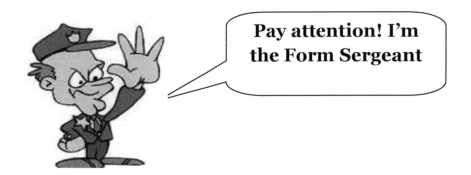

He will appear throughout the following pages to remind you of CORRECT postural and movement cues for each exercise!

Pay attention to the cues and begin to replace poor postural habits with an increased awareness of your body position especially when training to improve your balance and stability and prevent future falls.

After all, if you're going to put forth the effort to exercise, you want to make sure you're doing it right!!!

## GUIDELINES FOR BALANCE TRAINING

### 1.   Do balance training first

Balance involves the neuro-musculo-skeletal systems of the body.  In other words, your central nervous system is challenged during balance training.

I recommend practicing your balance exercises immediately after the warm-up when your body is fresh and your brain is alert.

### 2.  Practice balance training 3-4 times a week

Like any other motor skill, your balance will get better the more you practice.  Neural pathways will be formed and existing ones will fire more efficiently.

In other words, the body will respond to what the brain says quicker.

However, your body needs rest.  Growth and recovery happen on your days off so you want to give your body time to adapt to these new demands.

It is *recommended* (not required) that you try to practice some type of balance exercise three or four times a week for about 10 minutes each day.

### IT'S YOUR LIFE. LIVE IT!

Make the four types of exercise in a fall prevention program part of your lifestyle.

Make the time. 10 minutes a day.
It's your choice!

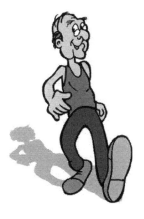

## 3. ALWAYS, ALWAYS, ALWAYS practice safety measures

- Chair in front and a wall behind you when standing
- Sturdy surface to onto
- Stop when you feel dizzy or short of breath
- Wear lightweight shoes and comfortable clothing
- Have your lifeline on or cell phone nearby
- Drink plenty of water
- Stop when you feel frustrated.  Enough is enough!

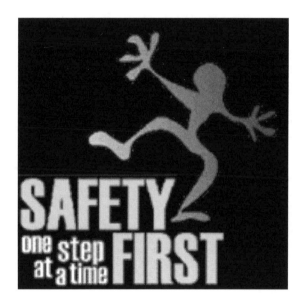

## PART II: DEMONSTRATE

### Fall Prevention Exercise Program

Following this program will challenge your balance, stretch and strengthen your body and improve your posture to reduce your risk of an accidental fall.

The types of exercises in this fall prevention exercise program include:

1. Postural awareness
2. Balance training 101™
3. Strength-building activities
4. Flexibility exercises
5. Endurance and Walking Gait training

**Congratulations!**

**You are now ready to begin your fall prevention exercise program**

**Have fun and be safe!!!**

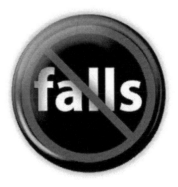

## Warm-Up

The purpose of the warm-up is to prepare the muscles, connective tissues, ligaments and joints for the work you're about to do.

Warm muscles are a lot more flexible than cold muscles so **ALWAYS** include some type of warm up before exercise.

```
Appropriate warm up exercises include:

Walking
Gentle stretching exercises
Total body calisthenics
```

## Proper Seated Position

Just like we have to be able to crawl before we can walk, it's good to start with the basics when starting a fall prevention exercise program, especially balance training. Good Form Starts While Seated!

If you haven't exercised in a while, it's important that you learn good movement patterns and how to do them safely. Once your body adjusts to the basics, you can increase the challenges.

The basics start in your chair. After you learn good habits while seated, you practice those same habits while standing and walking. Eventually good movement patterns can become part of your lifestyle.

I begin by having students get into what I call "proper seated position".

You can start at the ground and work your way up.

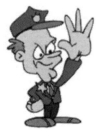

**Get in Proper Seated Position!**

## See the seated checklist below:

_____ 1. Both feet are on the floor, facing forward

_____ 2. Knees are slightly bent, facing forward

_____ 3. Hips are scooted to the back of the chair

_____ 4. Belly button is pulled in toward your spine

_____ 5. Lift your chest up toward the ceiling

_____ 6. Drop your shoulders down toward your back pockets

_____ 7. Chin is parallel to the floor

_____ 8. Tuck your chin in toward your neck

_____ 9. Ears are in line with your shoulders

_____ 10. Your eyes are focused on a vertical target at eye level

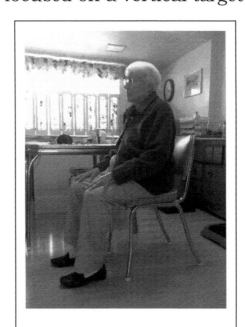

Proper Seated Position

## Sample Routine

Below is a *sample warm-up routine* that I use in my classes:

Neck Rotations:

- Sit tall, turn head to right, then center, then left, then center Repeat 5 times each direction.
- Find a vertical target each time you turn your head.

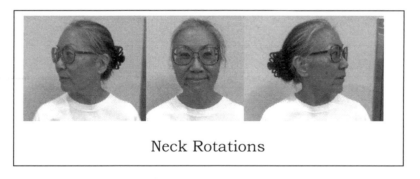

Neck Rotations

Shoulder Circles:

- Raise shoulders up toward ears then back and down in circular motion.
- Repeat 5 in one direction then do 5 shoulder rolls in opposite direction.

Arm Circles:

- Extend arms straight out to sides at shoulder height with thumbs up.
- Start moving arms in circular motion. Keep body still.
- Do 10 in forward direction then pause and repeat in backward direction.
- Start with small circles and slowly get bigger.

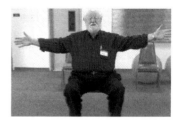

## Wrist Circles:

- Extend arms in front of body.
- Keep arm still as you draw circles with hands, working the wrist.
- Do 5 in one direction, pause and do 5 in opposite direction.

## Trunk Rotation:

- Put hands on thighs or crossed on chest.
- Exhale as you turn from the hip to look over right shoulder.
- Pause then return to center. Exhale and turn upper body to look over left shoulder.
- Keep shoulders level as you turn and try to look at wall behind you.
- Repeat 5 in each direction.

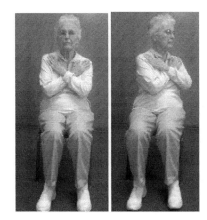

## Toe Taps (Seated or Standing)

- Both feet are flat on the floor.
- Extend right foot and tap toe to floor.
- Return to foot to start position then extend left foot and tap toe to floor.
- Repeat 10 times, alternating legs

## Heel Taps (Seated or Standing)

- Same exact exercise as above except you are tapping heel to the floor, not toe.
- Do 10 repetitions, alternating legs

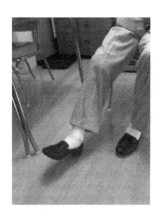

Side steps: (Seated or Standing)

Seated:

- Both feet on floor, alternate tapping toes out to side
- Right toe to right side, left toe to left side
- Repeat 10 times, alternating feet

Standing:

- Step right foot out to the right.
- Shift weight onto right foot then step over with left foot.
- Step left foot to the left, shift weight onto left foot then step over with right foot.
- Repeat 5 single side steps in each direction.
- Hold onto chair if you need to, keep chin parallel to the floor and eyes on vertical target.

Knee lifts:

- March in place behind chair
- Keep body tall, tighten stomach, lift knee, return to floor
- Tighten belly and bring knee up as high as you can without bending forward
- Tighten stomach, lift other knee.
- Repeat 10 times, each leg, alternating legs.

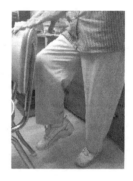

Knee Lifts

Butt kickers:

- March in place except you want to bring your heels as far up to your buttocks as you can.
- Squeeze muscle in back of leg to pull heel up toward butt.
- Do 10 each leg, alternating legs.

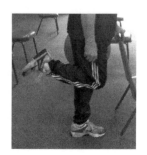

Butt Kickers

Stretch calves:

- Stand behind chair
- Step back with right foot and drop right heel to the floor
- Shift weight to front foot, keeping back leg straight and heel on the floor
- Bend front knee slightly as you shift weight forward
- Hold 10 seconds. Repeat with left leg.

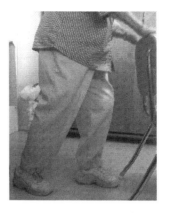

Calf Stretch

**Now your body is ready to do some balance training!**

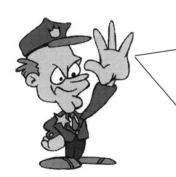

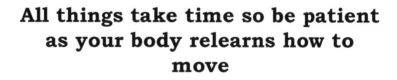

**NOTE:**

**If this warm up was difficult, just do the seated *portion until your body adapts the demands of exercise.***

**All things take time so be patient as your body relearns how to move**

# BALANCE TRAINING 101™ EXERCISES

## Introduction

First, please understand that balance is a motor skill and like any other motor skill, it can improve with practice. You may currently be engaged in a strength and stretching routine but do nothing to challenge your balance.

While standing on one leg or walking heel to toe are good balance exercises, there is more to balance training than those exercises. The balance training component of your program should be:

- Individualized to meet your needs
- Progressively challenging to allow continued improvement
- Training the muscles and senses involved in balance and mobility

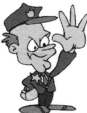

**DO NOT try a more challenging level until you feel confident doing the exercise at the easier level.**

## Individualized
- Know your limitations and push yourself according to your abilities.

## Progressions
- The three sensory systems that affect our balance are the:
  o Eyes
  o EARS
  o Feet

- To progressively challenge your balance alter the placement of:
  o Eyes
  o ARMS
  o Feet

1. **Eyes:**

   We rely heavily on vision for feedback about our balance.

In some exercises, it will be suggested that you close your eyes if you are ready.  Here are some visual progressions:

- Easiest:  Eyes open
- Moderate:  Wear dark sunglasses or read a large print poem
- Most challenging:  Eyes closed

2. **Arms:**
   Arm placement affects our balance.  Here are some arm progressions:

- Easiest:  Holding onto an external surface (Chair or counter)
   - 2 fingers on surface
   - Hover hands above surface
- Moderate:  Hands down by side or resting on lap
- Most challenging:  Arms crossed on your chest

3. **Feet:**

Your feet are your base of support.

Without getting too complicated, the wider your feet are apart, the steadier you feel.

- Easiest:  Feet hip-width apart
- Moderate:  Toes and heels together
- Challenging:  Split stance, Semi-tandem, Tandem, 1-leg

**These different foot placements will be discussed in the next section.**

## Postural Awareness

Remember when your parents and grandparents used to tell you:

- *"QUIT SLOUCHING"*
- *"STAND UP STRAIGHT"*
- *"PRETEND LIKE YOU HAVE A BOOK ON YOUR HEAD"?????*

Well, it turns out they were onto something really good!!!!

### The Benefits of Proper Alignment Include:

- Increased lung capacity therefore more oxygenation to body
- Less stress and strain on your skeletal frame, joints, and muscles
- Improved digestion due to organs in proper alignment
- Increased energy since your body doesn't have to work as hard

Good postural habits help prevent falls


### Remember the postural checklist, starting from the ground:

1. Both feet are on the floor, facing forward

2. Knees are slightly bent, facing forward

3. Hips are scooted to the back of the chair

4. Belly button is pulled in toward your spine

5. Lift your chest

6. Drop your shoulders

7. Chin is parallel to the floor

8. Tuck your chin in toward your neck

9. Ears are in line with your shoulders

10. Your eyes are focused on a vertical target at eye level

11. Pretend you have a string attaching your head to the ceiling to elongate your spine

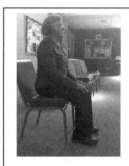

Correct
Seated
Posture

## Belly Button Training

*(Yay! Our belly button finally has a purpose!)*

**Balance is keeping your center of gravity over your base of support.**

**Translation: Keep your belly button over your feet.**

In the human body, the area around the belly button is referred to as our center of gravity (center of mass).

The placement of your feet is your base of support, whether you are standing still or moving.

With age, we move more from our head or feet and forget to take the belly button with us!

This may not make sense but if the majority of your mass is around the belly (like mine), it's important to learn how to move the body efficiently so that gravity is on your side!

**The goal of belly button training is to improve efficiency while you move through space or while standing still.**

First, I want you to start paying attention to where your belly button is in location to the rest of your body.

If you are like some of my clients, you are fighting "old-age posture" by keeping your shoulders back but unfortunately, this can throw your hips forward.

## Typical poor "Old age" posture:

- Chin jutted forward
- Eyes looking downward
- Shoulders rounded forward
- Curved spine; uneven shoulders
- Hips shifted backward
- Weight heavy on the heel

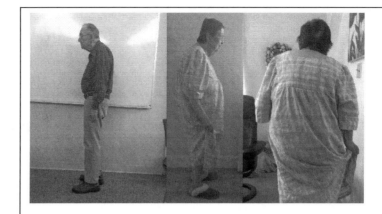

Common "Old age" postures

## Correctly aligned posture:

- Ears over shoulders
- Chin parallel to floor
- Eyes focused straight ahead
- Shoulders over hips & level
- Hips in line with ankles
- Weight between toes and heels

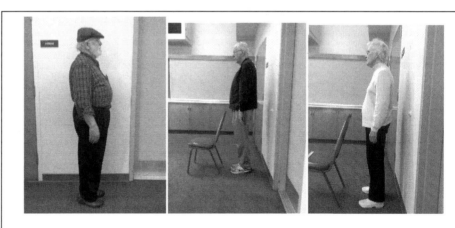

Correctly aligned postures

## Let's improve your posture!!!

---

### *Postural Checklist:*

- Both feet on the floor
- Knees are facing forward and are directly above ankles
- Belly pulled in toward spine
- Shoulders are aligned with hips
- Ears are directly above your shoulders
- Chin parallel to floor
- Eyes focused forward
- STRING attaching head to ceiling to elongate spine

---

## Seated Posture

- Get into proper seated position in the middle of your chair
- Pay attention to your body position in space
- Run the postural checklist through your mind
- Keep eyes open and focused on vertical target for 15-30 seconds

## Progressions:

- Eyes: Eyes open, dark glasses on, eyes closed
- Arms: On surface, down by sides, crossed on chest.

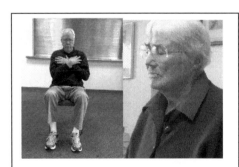

Cross Arms  Close eyes

# Tighten and Hold!!!  Tighten and Hold!!!

## (This Is A Must-Do Stabilizer Exercise)

We are breaking our backs.  Nearly 80% of Americans will experience low back pain at some point in their lives.

Weak stomach and deep postural muscles contribute to these back problems because they do not support and stabilize the spine.  An unstable spine can easily be "thrown out" of alignment.

### Balance is about being stable.

Luckily, we have a naturally built-in girdle (a deep postural muscle called the TVA) to stabilize the spine.  Without getting too scientific on you....listen to me...

### If you want to protect your back,

### you have to tighten the front!

You can do this simple exercise ANYTIME, ANYWHERE, especially while you are sitting down! Do it while waiting in the doctor's office or while watching TV.  Try it now!


### TIGHTEN AND HOLD EXERCISE

Seated:

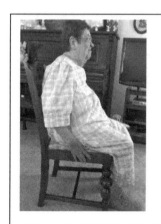

- Scoot your hips to the back of the chair so your back is in contact with the back of the chair
- Both feet are on firmly on the floor, chest is lifted and shoulders down
- TIGHTEN your stomach muscles as you pull belly button in toward spine
- Press your low back against the chair.  HOLD
- Keep shoulders back and down and chest lifted as you hold
- **TIGHTEN** stomach as you press low back against the chair and **HOLD** for 10 seconds.  Tighten, hold (10 seconds), Repeat 10 times

Do this seated then try **standing against a wall.**

When standing, TRY to get your entire body against the wall: heels, hips, shoulders, head. If you need to walk your feet out a step to do this, that's ok.

**Tighten the stomach, press low back against the wall, and HOLD!**

### Standing: Check Standing posture and Belly Button:

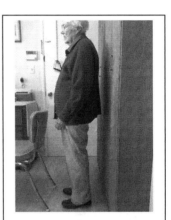

- Stand behind chair and **in front of a wall** (not touching or leaning against wall in this exercise) with feet hip-width apart
- Eyes are open and you are looking at <u>vertical target</u>.
- Hold this standing posture for 15-30 seconds being fully aware of the position of your body as you are standing still.
- Now close your eyes. Continue to run the postural checklist through your mind as you feel the pressure under your feet.
- Try to hold this stance for 15-30 seconds. Then try with eyes closed.

**You may feel yourself swaying but that is perfectly normal!**

**If you feel unsteady, open your eyes and grab the chair.**

---

### MILLION DOLLAR TIP: HOMEBASE

**Homebase** is the centered posture that I refer to.

**Homebase** is the center spot where your body is perfectly aligned.

It's when you feel the weight equally distributed under both feet and your ears, shoulders, hips, knees and ankles are in line.

**Homebase** is the space you come back to after an unexpected push, a quick stop, or an upper body turn. Your body comes back to center after reaching forward to put something on a shelf.

**Homebase** is comfortable. It's your resting posture. Your homebase is becoming perfectly aligned.

---

## Postural Exercise: Check Your Window

- With hands open wide, bring hands close to shoulders to form an imaginary window
- Stick your head out the window
- Then slide chin back as you bring head back in the window
- Sense that your ears are in line with your shoulders and keep chin parallel to floor
- Repeat 10 times

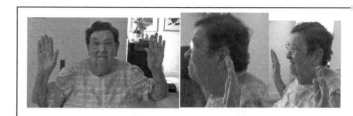

Form your window:  Out      In

**CHECK YOUR WINDOW**

### IS YOUR HEAD "OUT THE WINDOW" WHEN YOU:

- Drive your car?
- Sit at the computer?
- Walk down the street?

**Think about where you're carrying your head!**

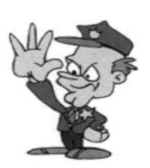

## Position of Feet:

Fall prevention is more than standing on one leg!

Balance is keeping the center of mass over the base of support whether moving or stationary (Rose, 2006). Your belly button area is your center of mass OR center of gravity. Your feet and the space between them is your base of support.

### Balance is keeping the belly button over the feet

As we age, weakened thigh and hip muscles make us unsteady. Practice these standing exercises and you will improve your balance and beat the "wobbly" feeling!

### Challenge # 1:  Position of Feet = Base of Support

You can do these exercises <u>while seated or standing</u>.  If you are seated, make sure you are in the middle of the chair.

If you are ready to try standing, make sure you stand behind a chair or sturdy surface and in front of a wall.

The placement of the feet in these pictures is from easiest to hardest. Add progressions when confident and ALWAYS be safe.

### Keep your knees slightly bent!

1. **Feet hip-width apart (EASIEST):**

- Stand tall with feet about as wide as your hips are apart
- Hold stance with eyes open and focused on a vertical target for 15-30 seconds
- TRY to close eyes, hold stance for 15-30 seconds

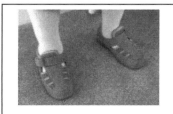

**Hip-width apart**

### **HOLD ONTO A SURFACE IF NEEDED**

## 2. Toes and heels together (1ˢᵗ CHALLENGE):

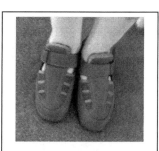

**Toes/Heels Together**

- Bring your heels and toes together so they are touching
- If you can't get toes AND heels together, just put HEELS together
- Stand tall, lift chest. Your chin is parallel to the floor and your eyes are focused on a vertical target
- Hold stance for 15-30 seconds

<u>Arm challenge:</u>  Can you hover hands above surface?  Hold on with 2 fingers?  One finger?  Put arms down by your sides?  The last arm challenge is arms crossed chest.

<u>Eye challenge:</u>  Try this stance with dark sunglasses on.  Can you try to close your eyes?  Hold stance for 15-30 seconds.

Standing like this may be more difficult than you think, especially with your eyes closed!  You may feel yourself swaying all over the place so start easy.

If it was easy with eyes open and arms crossed on chest, lower arms to side, then close eyes to see how you feel.

### DO NOT TRY THE FOLLOWING EXERCISES STANDING UNTIL YOU CAN MAINTAIN UPRIGHT POSITION WHILE SEATED

## 3. Split stance:

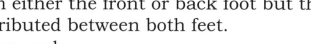

**Split Stance**

- Take one step forward with your right foot as if you were going to walk across the room.
- Make sure that the heel of the front foot is SOMEWHERE in front of the toe of the back foot.  This is not a narrow stance but more like a step.
- Shift weight so that you feel pressure under both feet.  In other words, not all your weight is resting on either the front or back foot but the weight is EQUALLY distributed between both feet.
- Hold stance for 15 - 30 seconds.

- Repeat with left foot in forward position

**Quick check....**At this point, if you were to drop a plumb line from your belly button to the floor, the line would land between your toe and heel. *(This is the only time I want you to look at the ground!)*

You're standing in split stance, your knees are slightly bent, your hips are level, your chest is lifted, shoulders are down, chin is parallel to the floor, eyes are focused on a vertical target

## INDIVIDUALIZED PROGRESSIONS in SPLIT STANCE

Obviously, there's a huge difference from taking a normal step forward and walking a tight rope. You would feel very unstable on a tight rope and that is because of weak hip muscles and poor balance skills.

Since you bought this book to help improve your balance, I want you to try this in the split stance:

**Inch your front foot over closer to the center of your body.** This may be 1 inch for some and it might be 3 inches for others.

I want you to inch that front foot over until <u>you</u> feel that's enough.

This is where you can practice and progress on your own. Your goal might be to stand on the tight rope one day. Or you might be ok standing on a 6-inch plank!

- Shift weight between your front and back foot, find the equal weight distribution spot (belly button between front heel and back toe)
- Look forward at vertical target. Lift chest. Drop shoulders.
- Add arm and eye challenges when ready.

Arms:

- Hold onto surface. 2 finger hold. Hover hands above surface. Arms down by side. Arms crossed on chest.
- Hold stance for 15 seconds with eyes open and arms placed where you feel safe.

- Then challenge your eyes when you are ready.

Eyes:

- Open focused on vertical target.  Dark glasses on.  Eyes closed.

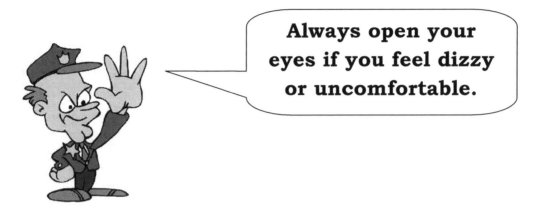

Always open your eyes if you feel dizzy or uncomfortable.

**I am not a doctor and this is not intended to diagnose you but if you have extreme dizziness with your eyes closed, you may have an inner ear disorder.**

**Tell your doctor or physical therapist about this situation.**

## ADVANCED:

These challenges are for the tight rope walkers!  **Only after** you have successfully been able to stand in a narrow split stance position without holding onto your surface should you to try this next stance.

Remember, as your feet get closer together like walking a tight rope, any weakness in your hips and legs plus lack of upper body postural control will become more evident.

### Semi-tandem:

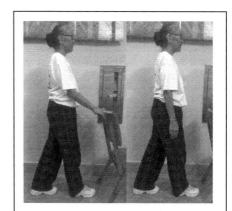

Semi-Tandem

- Starting in split stance, inch the front foot over as if you are balancing on a tight rope.
- Your front foot is directly in front of back foot but not touching it.
- A line from your belly button should drop between your heel and toe
- Eyes focused on a vertical target. Check your arm placement.  Hold for 15-30 seconds.
- Switch feet

DO NOT GIVE UP….you can get stronger with practice!

### Tandem:

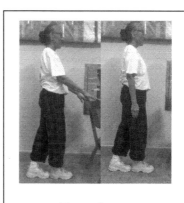

Tandem

- Slide the front foot back so that the front heel now touches the toes of the back foot.
- Imagine you are Heel to Toe on a tight rope
- Chest is lifted, shoulders are down. Eyes on a vertical target.  Check your arm placement.
- Hold for 15-30 seconds
- Switch feet
- If you have hardwood flooring, pick one rail to stand on and line feet up together.

## A Word of Caution:

These exercises may be much easier with one leg in front than the other due to prior injury or current weaknesses.

For instance, my left leg is definitely weaker than my right. As such, it is more difficult for me to do these exercises with my left foot forward.

Practice with both right and left leg in front.

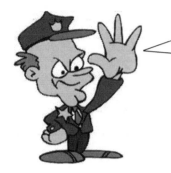

**Do not advance to the next level until you are able to complete the prior exercises SAFELY**

## One leg:

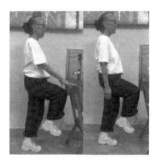

- Shift all your weight to right leg and lift the left foot off the ground
- Try to hold stance 15-30 seconds or as long as possible
- Repeat other leg

## PROGRESSIONS

I want to take the time and talk about these "progressions" before there is any confusion or feel like you can't do this. You can....if you work at <u>your</u> pace.

**These progressions are only suggestions, <u>not requirements.</u>**

With some foot placements, there is a huge difference between holding onto a surface and totally letting go.

That's ok, you can get more stable with practice.

YOU DO NOT HAVE TO LET GO of the surface!

When practicing the more narrow foot positions, you might want to try holding onto the surface with **two fingers.** This may be all you can do in some stances and THAT IS OK.

Eventually, you might want to try to let go of the surface but first, try to hover your hands above the surface.

When ready, put arms down by sides.

DO NOT attempt to cross your arms if you are unsteady or frightened.

These are suggestions ONLY.

You can also do something with your eyes. You can keep them open and focused on a vertical target.

Or you can put on some dark sunglasses or shut the curtains.

When closing your eyes for the first time with feet in a more narrow position, <u>put your hands back onto the surface</u> to make sure you are ok.

**<u>TRY COMBINATIONS:</u>** Change the placement of your feet, do something with your arms, then practice with eyes closed.

## *"It Makes Sense"* ™ Balance Training

To remain balanced, we rely on input from three (3) of our senses. There are different ways to challenge these senses but this usually requires specialized equipment.

I don't expect you to spend $200 on a stability ball, stability ball holder, dyna-disc, or Airex-pads so I will make sensible substitutions.

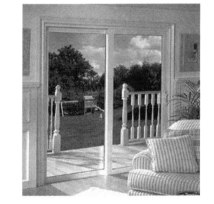

### Eyes (Visual Sensory Input)

Vision: we rely on visual input about the environment and our body position in space as it relates to balance.

Focus: Eyes on vertical target: One of the key components of the *FallProof*™ balance and mobility training program is to keep your eyes focused on a vertical target.

**Example of a vertical target**

According to feedback from class participants, looking at a vertical target is also one of the most helpful balance training techniques in the program.

A vertical target is:

- Eye level
- Stationary
- Directly in front of you

BENEFITS of looking at a vertical target:

- Gives your body a sense of stability when you are moving
- Increases stability when you turn your head
- Orients "old-age" posture to true vertical causing a person to sit taller
- Increases awareness of proper posture

## Eye Training

Yes, we need to train our eyes with respect to walking and fall prevention especially as we get older.

I call it "DEFENSIVE WALKING" or a way to improve your visual skills by looking around, up, and down while standing still or moving.

**I am NOT telling you to ignore the surface below you and just stare at your vertical target.**

Our eyes have muscles and those muscles enable us to dart the eyes down, up, to the right, to the left without moving the head.

To do this, check out the exercises below.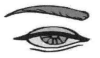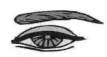

## Exercise 1: Pencil training

<u>Field of vision:</u> in this exercise, picture a box in front of your face. The box is about 12" x 12".

- Move the pencil within that box.
- Right to Left.
- Top to bottom.
- Diagonal; upper right to lower left and upper left to lower right.

**Slow eye movement:** use one pencil

Right to Left:

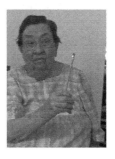

- Sit tall and keep your head still
- Follow the pencil through your field of vision (Pencil is moving slowly)
- Move pencil from right to left, then left to right
- Pause and check for dizziness. If dizzy, stop immediately. If ok, repeat for 10 seconds

Up and Down:

- Wait 10 seconds
- Put pencil in other hand

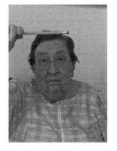

- Slowly move the pencil up to top of field of vision box
- Pause, then move pencil down through your field of vision
- Repeat 10-20 seconds

Diagonal

- Slowly move pencil down to lower left corner
- Pause, check for dizziness
- Repeat lower left to upper right for 10-20 seconds.
- Put pencil in opposite hand and repeat diagonals, this time upper left corner to lower right. Keep head still!

**Fast eye movement:** 2 pencil training

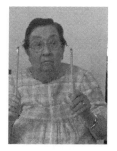

Right/Left

- Hold a pencil in each hand about 6-8 inches apart
- Without moving head, dart your eyes as fast as you can from right to left, looking at the pencil in each hand each time
- Repeat for 10 seconds then pause

Up/Down

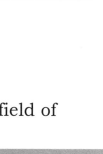

- Hold two pencils above each other about 6-8 inches apart. Do not move head as you look at pencil in top hand then bottom hand as quickly as you can.
- Find the pencil eraser each time
- Repeat for 10 seconds
- Pause 30 seconds before going onto next activity

Diagonal:

- Hold one pencil in the upper right corner of your field of vision box and the other pencil in the lower left corner, about 8-10 inches apart.
- Quickly and without moving your head, look at the pencil in upper right then lower left.

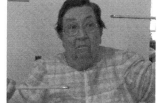

- Repeat as fast as you can for 10 seconds. Pause.
- Switch hands so now upper left and lower right and keep eyes still as you look between pencils as fast as you can.

### Great job!

Remember, the eyes have muscles & those muscles need to be worked.

Progressions while pencil training:

1. Bring your feet closer together
2. Sit on a thick cushion, dyna-disc, or stability ball
3. Try this activity while standing

## Feet (Scientific Term: Somatosensory)

We have feelers (or body position receptors) under our feet that give us feedback about our body, the environment, and how both relate to our balance.

As we get older, we lose the ability to feel our feet in contact with the ground. As a result of this reduced sensation, we sway more while standing still so our body can recognize where we are in space. Cool, huh?

Not so cool if you have peripheral neuropathy or nerve damage in the feet and legs and you can't feel the ground at all.

The *purpose of this portion* of "It Makes Sense" balance training is to *increase the awareness* of how far you can <u>lean while seated</u> or <u>shift while standing</u> without losing your balance.

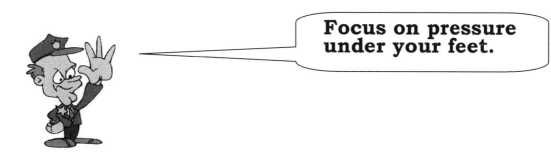

**Focus on pressure under your feet.**

# All exercises are done with sunglasses on, lights dimmed or eyes closed.

If you can't close your eyes and do the exercises, do not get discouraged. Try the sunglasses while doing the following activities.

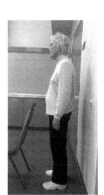

### Exercise 1: Feel pressure under feet

- Sit or stand in proper position. Homebase. Feet are hip-width apart.
- Eyes are closed or you have sunglasses on
- **Feel the pressure under your feet**
- Weight should be equally distributed between both feet and between heels and toes.

Check arm placement: On the surface, hover above, 2 fingers touching, down by side, or crossed on chest.

Hold stance, focusing on pressure under your feet for 15-30 seconds.

Now try changing the placement of your feet.

Concentrate on the pressure under your feet as you try these different stances:

a. Toes and heels together

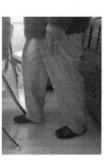

b. Split Stance

**Remember that in order to fully use the senses in your feet, you must do something with your eyes!**

**(Close them, wear dark sunglasses, read a poem)**

### Exercise 2: Seated Trunk Leans

"Grandpa, could you pass the turkey?" "Grammy, Santa missed that present behind your chair", "Auntie, could you grab my socks out of the dryer?" "Honey, it's your turn to unload the dishwasher".....

Regardless of physical capability (or lack thereof), these are common situations in everyday life when you must be able to control your upper and lower body in order to prevent a fall.

This postural control starts in the seated position and begins with Trunk Leans. The "trunk" is the area above your hips, from the hips to the shoulders.

Throughout your balance training and LIFE, you want to keep your trunk upright and in good posture with your head and neck.

After all, you need to be able to pass the turkey at Thanksgiving without falling out of your chair, right?

You need to be able to pass Christmas gifts to your grandchildren without falling out of the chair, correct?

You don't want to strain your back when you grab socks out of the dryer and you definitely don't want to fall while doing your "honey-do" list. Right? Right.

**Exercise guidelines for seated trunk leans:**

- Body rotates from the hip. Pay attention to the pressure under your feet as you do these exercises.
- Pretend you are in the middle of a clock; 12 o'clock is in front of you and 6 o'clock is behind you.
- Sit tall in your chair, in proper seated position

**Sit <u>far enough forward</u> in your chair so that you can feel your feet in contact with the ground**

- Put your arms where you feel comfortable
- Put on dark sunglasses, dim the lights or close your eyes

<u>Forward Action:</u>

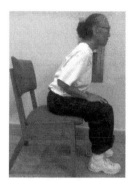

Forward Trunk Lean

- Keeping your body tall and upright, lean forward to 12 o'clock
- Focus on feeling the pressure increase under your feet shifting to your toes as you lean forward from the hip. Hold at the forward position for 3 seconds
- Tighten belly and return to start (homebase)
- Repeat forward trunk lean 5 times, hold 3 seconds at forward position before returning to "homebase"

Pretend you have a wooden plank strapped to your back. It extends from your tailbone to above your head. It's as wide as your back and it's tied to you.

- When you lean forward, your upper body stays as straight as the plank
- No rounding forward. You hinge forward and backward from the hip

If you do not feel the pressure increase under your feet, try scooting your hips forward so you are sitting more toward the front of the chair. Do not lean against the back of the chair in this exercise!

**<u>Trunk Lean Reminders:</u>**

- Keep dark glasses on or eyes closed throughout the movement
- Focus on pressure under feet as you lean forward
- Feel tension increase in thighs as you lean forward
- Keep upper body tall

Next, you are going to <u>lean backward toward 6 o'clock.</u>

Because a lot of older adults are TERRIFIED of leaning in the backward direction, you may want to start with your hands on your lap to feel your hands slide on your thighs as you lean backward.

Backward Trunk Lean:

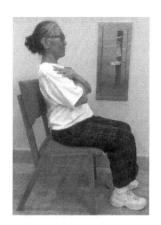

- Keep body tall and lean back as if going toward 6'clock
- Feel the pressure shift to your heels and your belly tighten as you lean back
- Keep your shoulders down
- Hold for 3 seconds.  Return to homebase.
- Feel the pressure shift from heels to center of foot.
- Repeat backward trunk lean 5 times

## DO NOT LEAN TOO FAR BACK!!!

## KEEP FEET ON THE FLOOR!!!!

This exercise requires control of upper body. Your stomach and lower back muscles must keep your spine stable as you move.

Weak muscles cannot support your upper body moving large distances. START SLOWLY.

- Shift weight to buttock as you gently lean backward, feeling angle at hip get larger.
- Your stomach muscles will tighten up. That is normal.
  Do not lean too far back. Stop when you feel the feet coming off the ground.
- Front to back, without stopping at homebase
- Sit tall in middle of chair
- Feet firmly on the floor
- Dark glasses on, lights dimmed or eyes closed

Front To Back, Without Stopping At Homebase

- Sit tall in middle of chair
- Feet firmly on the floor
- Dark glasses on, lights dimmed or eyes closed

Action:

- Lean forward toward 12 o'clock, feel pressure increase under balls of feet and feel tension in your thighs. Hold 3 seconds.
- Gently lean back toward 6 o'clock. Feel the pressure shift from toes to your heels. Or you may feel the lightness under your feet as your belly muscles tighten as you lean backward.
- Hold 3 seconds
- Repeat 5 times. Feel the pressure shift under your feet from toes to heels as you lean front to back

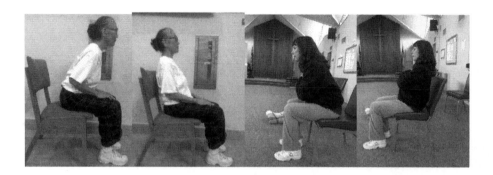

---

### **Progressions:**

Where are your arms?
- Down by sides
- Crossed on chest

Where are your feet?
- Toes/Heels together
- Split stance

**EYES ARE CLOSED**

---

## Trunk turns to the sides

For those of us still driving, we all have them; the dreaded blind spots.

Doing these trunk turns to the sides help you to check those spots without driving off the road.

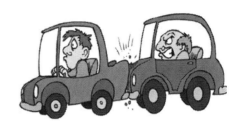

These are the same trunk rotations that you do in the warm up except now you are paying attention to the pressure under your feet while you do the exercise.

Right And Left Side Rotations:

- Sitting tall with eyes closed and arms in challenging position
- Inhale then exhale as you turn from the hip to look over your right shoulder.
- Feel the pressure under your left foot and tension in your left thigh as you do this turn to the right   Hold 3 seconds then return to homebase.
- Repeat 5 times to the right then do 5 times to the left.

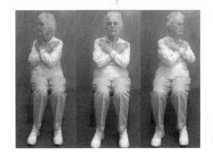

The goal is look at the wall behind you.  Your sternum (breastbone) should be facing toward the side that you are turning (see diagram).

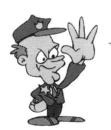

**Keep body tall.  Exhale as you turn away from homebase.  Inhale as you return.  Keep shoulders level.**

**FEEL THE PRESSURE UNDER THE OPPOSITE FOOT AS YOU TURN YOUR TRUNK TO THE SIDE**

**How can I look for a vertical target if my eyes are closed?**

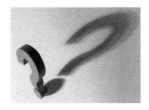

That's easy! Pretend the vertical target is tattooed on the inside of your eyelids! Envision the same vertical target you were looking at with your eyes open but now, it's on the inside of your eye lids!

### Inner Ear (scientific Term:  VESTIBULAR)

The inner ear mechanism plays a vital role in our balance.  The balance part of the inner ear is not the same as the hard of hearing inner ear.  Wearing hearing aids does not affect your balance the way an inner ear disorder does.

We rely on this system for balance when the other senses (eyes and feet) are distracted or impaired.  For instance, you cannot see well at night.  You also cannot feel the ground under your feet so well when you walk across the yard.

*Walk across the yard at night,* you are relying on your inner ear for input about your balance.  Do it in high heels and rely on the Almighty one to get you across!

Please be cautious with the following exercises if you:

- Ever had vertigo or vertigo-like symptoms.
- Have been diagnosed with Meniere's disease
- Been treated with chemotherapy drugs that bring on vertigo-like symptoms

If you get dizzy when you turn your head, you may have an inner ear disorder.

Some inner ear problems are temporary and others are permanent.  I suggest making an appointment with a physical therapist to have this type of condition checked out.  Look for a vestibular specialist or a referral from your ear, nose and throat doctor.

### Inner Ear Training:

These seated exercises require you to put something underneath your feet and if possible, something soft to sit on. Use a towel folded in half, an old patio seat cushion, foam pad, dyna-disc or stability ball.

AND your eyes should be closed or wear some dark sunglasses!

Let's start with some exercises.

## "Sense" body position in space

Seated Posture:

- Pad or cushion under feet and buttocks. Eyes closed or glasses on.
- Sit tall in the middle of your chair (say good-bye to the back of your chair, again)
- Think about postural cues (think postural checklist)
- Close your eyes. Please note: there is no movement at this time so try to close the eye. However if you feel unsafe, put on a pair of dark sunglasses.
- Hold this position for 15-30 seconds as you sense your body position in space

Exercise 1: Seated arm raises

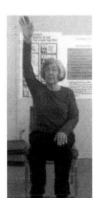

Single arm:

- Sitting on pillow or cushion with eyes closed, place feet on towel or patio cushion
- Raise right arm as far up as you can
- Hold for 3 seconds then lower
- Repeat 5 times right arm then 5 times with left arm

Both arms:

- Exhale as you raise both arms overhead.
- Keep upper body tall, chest lifted
- Shoulders over hips
- Pause at top for 3 seconds

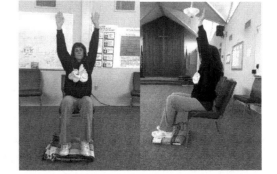

- Lower to start
- Repeat 5 times

Do NOT lean back as you raise your arms!!!

### Word of caution:

Due to shoulder limitations and prior injuries, you may not be able to raise one arm (or both) very far.

DO NOT exceed your limits.

Keep body tall and lift as high as you can without changing your upper body position.

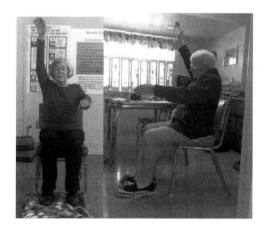

Exercise 2: Marching With Head Turns:  Can be done seated or standing!!!

Each time you turn your head and eyes, you activate the inner ear balance system.

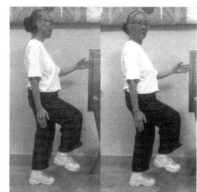

**The purpose of this exercise** is to be able to turn the head while marching without getting dizzy <u>and</u> without turning the upper body.  This can prevent a fall while you are window shopping, grocery shopping or crossing a busy intersection.

- March in place behind chair, looking forward at vertical target
- Count 6 steps, then turn head only to the right, finding a new vertical target
- March 6 strides, then turn head back to center
- Count 6 then turn head to left
- Turn head: center, right, center, left.  Counting for 6 counts before turning
- Repeat for 30 seconds

## Challenges

- Try to let go of the surface you are holding onto
- Lower number of counts to 4
- Turn head without pausing at center.
- Find a different vertical target each time
- March on thick pad or carpet.

**Pick up feet.  Lift knees.**

**Stop if you get dizzy or short of breath.**

**Try not to turn shoulders as you turn head.**

## Reaction Strategies

Think about this...the <u>ankle is the first joint</u> that must **react** to an uneven walking surface.

If you are walking and step on a cracked, uneven piece of sidewalk and you don't have any flexibility or strength in your ankle, your likelihood of falling is pretty good.

Bet you didn't know.....

Between the ages of 55-80, women lose over half and men lose over a third of their ankle flexibility?

And that the **reaction time** of a 60-year old CAN BE **25% slower** than a 20 year old.

<u>Solution</u>: Do ankle circles, toe point and flex and practice this reaction strategy!

## Ankle Reaction Strategy

The purpose of this training is to learn how far you can lean forward and backward without losing your balance. For this exercise....

- Pretend your entire body is stiff as a board (<u>cannot bend at waist</u>)
- Your feet are concreted to the ground (<u>cannot lift toes or heels</u>)

### Forward Ankle Leans:

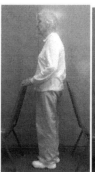
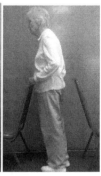

- Stand with feet hip-width apart between 2 chair
- Shift weight forward to your toes (do not bend at waist)
- Keep heels on ground as you feel your belly/thigh touch the front chair.
- Hold for 3 seconds the return to homebase
- Repeat forward direction 5 times, holding for 3 seconds with pressure under toes

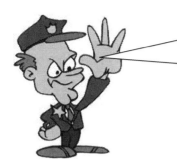

Keep toes and heels on the floor!

Do NOT just bend forward...feel belly button tap chair

This next exercise might be scary for some people so you do NOT have to attempt this exercise if you don't want to.

## Backward Ankle Leans:

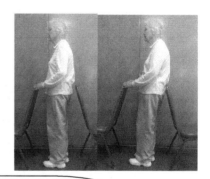

- Stand with feet hip-width apart
- Shift weight to heels
- Feel buttock tap chair or wall
- Hold for 3 seconds
- Shift weight to balls of feet (homebase)
- Repeat 5 times, shifting weight to heels and lightly tapping chair with buttocks

**KEEP TOES ON GROUND**

**and**

**KEEP SHOULDERS DOWN!**

Pretend your body is dipped in starch!

## Front to Back Ankle Leans (DO NOT STOP AT HOMEBASE)

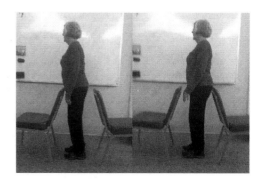

- Stand tall with feet hip-width apart
- Pretend body is dipped in starch and feet are rooted into ground
- Shift weight to toes. Hold 3 seconds
- Shift weight to heels. Hold 3 seconds
- Repeat 10 times without stopping at homebase.
- Keep toes and heels in contact with floor the entire time

**The distance you are able to shift your weight while keeping your feet on the ground is directly related to your ankle strength and flexibility.**

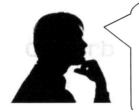

Do NOT think that these have to be big leans!!!

These are subtle shifts and your feet remain in contact with the floor.

## Common Mistakes:

1. Bending forward at waist
   Correction:
   - Shift weight to toes and bring belly button forward with you
   - Tap chair with belly button
   - Keep upper body stiff

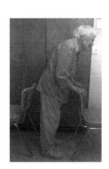

2. Leading backward with head or shoulders
   Correction:
   - Shift weight to heels
   - Tap butt against chair
   - Keep shoulders down and eyes forward

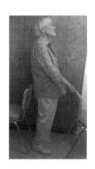

Progressions during Ankle leans

- Arm placement
  - On surface
  - 2 fingers on surface
  - Hover above surface
  - Down by sides
  - Crossed on chest
- Eyes (Open, Dark glasses, closed)
- Shift front to back quicker (don't hold as long)
- STEP OUT FROM BETWEEN CHAIRS

## Strength Training

Adults need lean muscle mass to remain independent.  In order to build or maintain muscle mass, you need to overload the muscles. Simply, you must put some effort into it and push or pull harder than it feels possible (fatigue), especially the 4 last repetitions of an exercise.

### Proper form

The important thing is not to lose proper form.  It's probably because my father was a Brigadier General in the Marines but I'm a "proper-form Sergeant".

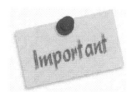

I am a stickler for doing exercises correctly in order to get the most benefit from your efforts.  Efficient movement?  Educated trainer?  Control freak? Definitely the first two....

I have cues and pictures for you to see how to properly perform an exercise.

Pay attention to your form and stop if you feel like you can no longer maintain form while doing the exercise.  That's how people get hurt.

### Don't forget to Breathe!

That's right; the cells need oxygen for energy.  Every little cell needs oxygen, even all the way down to the cells in your pinky toes!

## The rule of breathing while building muscle is to exhale on exertion

Examples of correct breathing….

When getting up from a chair, do you inhale or exhale as you stand up?

The correct answer is you should exhale as you stand up and inhale as you sit down.

Exhale as you pick up the grocery bag from the car trunk, exhale as you put down on the counter. And don't forget to breathe while carrying the bag in from the car!

**When** **you exert the most effort** **is when you need to blow out.**

## Warm UP

Always, always warm up, especially before doing strength-building exercises because the ligaments, tendons and connective tissue that surround and support the muscles are less likely to be injured if blood is circulating to muscles.

## Exercise order

Big muscles first! Hips, legs, back, chest. Those muscles require the most blood and burn the most calories when worked (calorie is a source of energy and big muscles need energy to function).

You want to keep the big muscles strong in order to reduce the risk of a fall.

**The number one cause of falls is**

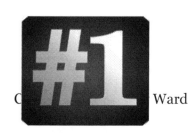

C                    Ward

# LOWER BODY WEAKNESS

American Council on Sports Medicine guidelines:

Allow 48-72 hours between resistance training sessions.

Your body needs time to recover.

I'm not talking about getting up out of the chair exercises but those movements that you use dumbbells or a resistance band.

### *"Muscles aren't built in the gym; they're built on your day off"*

---

**WHY CAN'T I BUILD MUSCLE EVERYDAY?**

When you push yourself to build muscle, you are causing tears within the muscle at microscopic level.  The <u>inflammation police come in and repair</u> by building leaner, stronger muscle.

That is how you get stronger.  This process takes anywhere between 48 and 72 hours.

And the older you get, the longer the recovery.

Stretch during this time, drink plenty of water and you should be feeling back to normal and ready to try again in 2 or 3 days.

If the recovery period is longer than four or five days, you may have overdone it or injured yourself.

**<u>Pay attention to your body!</u>**

---

# STRENGTHENING EXERCISES

## Hips

Weak hip muscles contribute to instability or the feeling of unsteadiness many people feel. The outer hip muscles weaken with age and the inner thigh muscles get tight. This muscular imbalance is common among older, sedentary individuals.

I recommend strengthen the outer thigh muscles and stretching the inner ones.

This is not a weight loss program however if you want to lose that flabby skin on your inner thigh, tightening ALL the thigh muscles will be helpful.

Most of these exercises can be done without any equipment but there are some exercises that require a resistance band, dumbbells or soup cans.

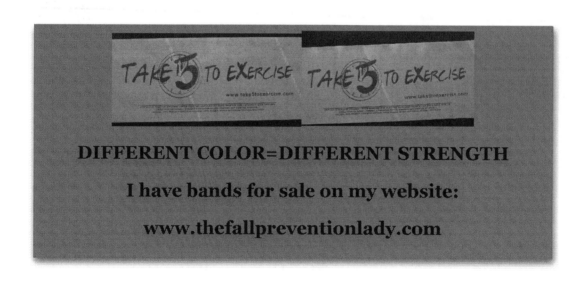

**DIFFERENT COLOR=DIFFERENT STRENGTH**

**I have bands for sale on my website:**

**www.thefallpreventionlady.com**

## 1. Clam:  order your resistance band

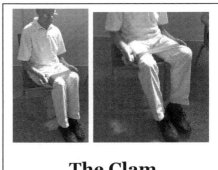

- Feet together, wrap band above knees so you're holding the ends of the band in each hand.
- Keep feet together as you open knees as far apart as possible (Roll ankles outward & keep feet on floor.
- Pause when knees are apart.
- Slowly close knees together, then open wide.  Pause. Start/Stop position is with knees open.
- Repeat 10-15 times.

**The Clam**

### IMPORTANT

Do these movements slow and controlled.

You are NOT mindlessly swinging the leg back and forth

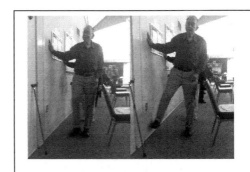

## 2. Foot to Wall

- Stand arms length away from the wall with arm outstretched to wall.
- Stand tall and shift weight to outer foot as you lift the inner leg toward the wall.

**Heel to Wall**

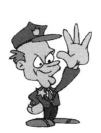

If you have to twist your body to get your heel to touch the wall, please step in closer to the wall.

It is important that you maintain proper posture to work the hip muscles.

At this point, **your body should be straight and properly aligned** (ears over shoulders, shoulder over hip and outer hip is over the ankle).

Belly button is pulled in tight and chin is parallel to the floor.

The knee of the leg that you're standing on is slightly bent.

### Action:

- Start/stop position is with heel touching the wall.
- Slowly lower heel toward the floor but do not touch the floor
- Exhale and return heel to wall.
- Touch the wall with your heel, not your toe
- Repeat 10-20 times.  Face the opposite direction and repeat with the other leg.

### Bonus action:

Pulse your heel against the wall 10-20 times.

(Pulse means do not lower heel more than 3 inches off the wall)

## *Where did you feel that?*

When you do the heel to wall correctly, you feel fatigue <u>in the hip of the leg you're standing on</u>, not the leg you are tapping against the wall.

## Legs/Calves/Ankles

The following exercises are what I call Beat the Wobbly moves because they strengthen the "fall prevention muscles" (your hips and thighs!!

I want you to try to do these exercises everyday and feel your lower body getting stronger.

Chair Stand:

By far the easiest, cheapest way to remain strong and independent is to get up out of your chair! If the chair is too low, you might want to practice getting up off the toilet because whether you know it or not, your legs are more likely to be in proper form when you're getting off the john!

Preparation:

- Place chair near wall if you are unsteady
- Sit in the middle of the chair.
- Make sure ankles are below your knees and feet are hip width apart. Keep chin parallel to floor and DO NOT LOOK AT THE FLOOR
- Hand placement makes this exercise progressively challenging

Action:

- Tighten belly and squeeze buttock as you stand up
- Come up to "homebase"; lifting your chin and chest upward as you drop your shoulders
- Feel the weight equally distributed between both feet, centered in the middle of your foot.
- Pause
- Slowly lower your hips toward the back of the seat for a count of 1, 2, 3, 4
- Repeat 5-20 times in a row, depending on your fitness level.

## Some people need to use their hands to get up!

That's ok!!!

Having to use your hands to get up is no excuse NOT to practice your chair stands!!! In fact, if you use your hands, you need to practice getting up even more!

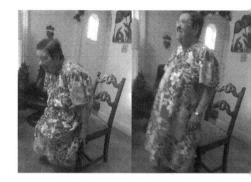

Yes, it's going to take effort. Exercise takes effort. Being strong and alive takes effort. Life wasn't intended to be easy. You have to try. Put forth an effort. Just do it.

I suggest using your hands to get up but still try to control how you sit down. Pause, then get back up again. And again. And again. You will get stronger!

---

### Story:

I have a client who uses her hands to get up. Partially be        ear of falling, she will not stand up unless she can use her h    Let's deal with that.

I have her do 10 chair stands using her hands.   She bar   mean barely, uses her hands to get up so I ask her to do 10 more.  She does 10 more.  This woman used to only be able to do 5 chair stands using her hands.  Now she can do 3 sets of 10 chair stands, using her hands.

At some point along the way, her legs have gotten getting stronger!

Her form is beautiful and her nose takes off down the runway each time.

---

How you sit back down is as important as how you get up because you have to use muscles to lower yourself down, too.

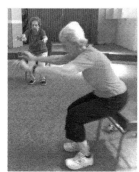

I see a lot of people do the "drop and flop"; just hoping the chair catches them as they free fall toward the seat.

Rather, I want you to slowly lower your hips toward the back of the seat for a count of 1, 2, 3, 4. You are bending your knees and reaching back with your hips/butt as you sit down.

---

**I TELL PEOPLE TO ENVISION THE WORST PORTA-POTTY EVER......**

**You know, the one where you're terrified to sit on the seat. Even fearful of what may come out from the depths below!!!**

**Lead with your hips as you sit down. Do this and you build strength and also protect your knees.**

---

### Set a personal goal number of chair stands to do each day

This is where individualized attention is important. Not everyone can get out of the chair 10 times in a row. Getting up 5 times may be a personal best for one person while it may not even phase another.

This is why I recommend doing the chair stand as an assessment test to measure where you are right now.

Then try to set a personal goal.

Follow this program, do your chair stands, then test again.

Your body will improve!

## Butt Kickers

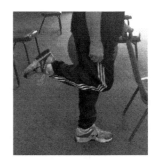

- Prep:  Stand behind a chair
- Action:  March in place, bending at the knee as you try to kick your heels toward your butt.
- Return to floor.
- Alternate feet, squeezing the muscle in the back of your leg to pull your heel toward your butt.
- Duration:  10-20 repetitions each leg or time yourself for 30 seconds

You may feel a stretch in the front of your leg when you do this exercise and that is normal. As you strengthen the muscles in the back of your leg, you stretch the muscles in the front

## Toe Raises: (done seated or standing)

- Prep:  Sit in a chair or stand behind chair
- Action:  shift weight to heels as you lift toes off the ground
- Return toes to floor.
- Duration:  Repeat lifting toes as high as you can off the floor 10-20 times or during commercial breaks. I recommend starting in a seated position and then do these standing.

Feel the contraction in the front of lower leg.

## Exercise takes effort!  Make the effort!

If you have peripheral neuropathy, this exercise may be extremely difficult.  Please start out seated and try shifting the weight to your heels to raise the toes.  While standing, try to tap one foot at a time. Do 10 toes raises with the right foot, then 10 toe raises with the left, then 10 with both.

This is a must do if you want to prevent dragging your toes when you walk.  Great exercises you can do while watching TV, eating a meal, while waiting at the doctors, standing in line at grocery store.  These can be done anytime, anywhere.  Just shoot for 10 minutes at a time.

## Heel Raises (Go onto Tip-toes):

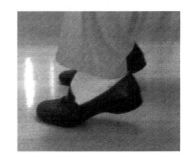

- Prep:  Sit in chair or stand behind chair
  Action: shift weight to balls of feet and lift heels off the floor.
  Feel the contraction in your calves (muscles in the back of lower leg)
- Repeat 10-20 times, during commercial breaks, at meals, while waiting, anytime, anywhere exercise.

## Toe point and flex:

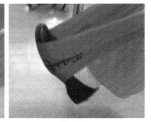

- Grab ends of resistance band in both hands
- Secure resistance band around right foot
- Extend right left keep leg extended.
- Point your toes away from your body
- Then flex as you pull toes toward body and push heel away.
- Repeat 15 times right foot then do 15 repetitions with left foot

## Flexion and Extension

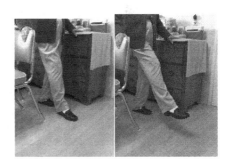

- Stand beside chair or sturdy surface
- Shift weight to left foot and extend right leg in front of body
- Tighten stomach and lift right leg off the ground.  Keep weight on left foot.
- Slowly lower leg to floor, tap ground and lift leg upward again.  Repeat 5-20 times.

*Now the tough part.....*

- After doing forward leg lifts, extend right leg behind body.
- Tighten stomach and squeeze right buttock to lift right leg off the ground.
- Lower toe toward ground (**tap toe, tighten stomach, squeeze buttock**) and raise right leg off the ground.  Keep weight on left foot.
- Repeat 5-15 times right leg.  Repeat same sequence with left leg.

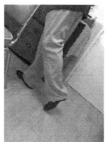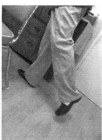

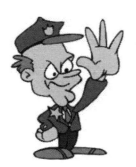

**Do not bend at the knee!!!**

**We did butt kickers earlier so for this exercise, you want to keep your leg straight.**

Postural cues:

- Keep leg straight.
- Keep upper body straight; do not bend forward to raise leg.
- When doing backward leg lifts, keep hips and shoulders facing forward.
- Try not to tilt forward.

This is an exercise for a muscle that doesn't get much use and may be very difficult to do at first.

## Back

**Seated Row:** GREAT FOR POSTURE!!!

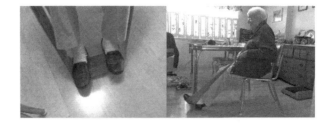

- Scoot to edge of chair and secure band around both feet.
- Pull band toward body as you keep your chest lifted, shoulders down and chin tucked back.  This is your start/stop position.
- Extend arms forward then pull back.   Exhale as you pull backward.
- Pause as you focus on pulling shoulders blades together
- Repeat 10-15 times

### 1-arm DB row: soup can or light dumbbell needed

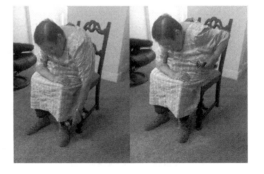

- Sit in chair, bend forward at waist and rest left elbow across knees.
- Right arm is holding soup can, water bottle or dumbbell down by toes
- Tighten stomach as you pull right arm back toward right arm pit.
- PAUSE, Squeeze armpit muscle (yes, you have one)
- Then lower the right arm back toward front of foot the ground.
- Repeat 10-15 times.

Postural reminders:  Keep shoulders level, back straight, and use the opposite arm to rest on knees.  This resting arm supports your lower back so use it so you don't hurt yourself in bent over position. Keep elbow close to your body as you pull back toward armpit.

## Chest

**Chest press:** (resistance band needed)

- Wrap band around body at armpit level
- Grab ends of band with hands and knuckles s facing forward
- Sit tall in the middle of the chair
- Exhale as you extend arms forward at chest level.
- Pause then slowly bring hands back toward shoulders. That is one repetition.
- Repeat 10-15 times.

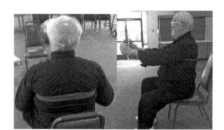

**Chest stretch:** The chest muscles are tight. Tight chest muscles pull your shoulders forward. This is why I recommend all my clients do this chest stretch. Daily.

- Grab your resistance band and wrap band around palms so hands are about shoulder width apart.
- Extend arms in front of you then exhale as you extend arms overhead.
- Inhale then exhale as you extend straightened arms overhead
- Pause. Inhale then exhale as you reach further back with straighten arms
- Hold 10-15 seconds
- Inhale and return arms to start position

Arms will tend to drop out toward side but try to keep tension in band (Do not pull apart). You will feel a tremendous stretch in the front of your shoulders.

Do this stretch slowly.

---

**Resistance band rules:**

1. Shorten distance between hands if exercise is too easy

2. Always keep tension on the band.

3. Slow and controlled movements

You are in control of the band

Remember…good form = good movement.

---

## Shoulders

### Horizontal pull

- Grab ends of resistance band a little more than shoulder width apart with arms extended in front of body.
- Keep chest lifted and shoulders down as you bring arms back, pinching shoulder blades together.
- SLOWLY bring hands back to start position. Do not just "let go" but control the band and stop when back to starting position. Do not allow slack in the band.
- Repeat 8-12 times

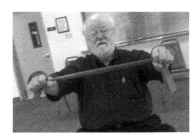
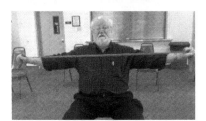

### Open the Refrigerator Door

- Sit tall, arms bent at 90 degrees at sides
- Tuck elbows into sides directly below shoulder (you may want to put a towel between your elbow and side).

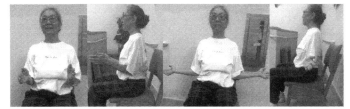

- Pretend you are opening refrigerator door as you open arm to side and backward as far as you can.
- Keep elbows against side and return to start
- Repeat, without weight 20-30 times
- You can do one arm at a time or both arms at the same time

## Pendulum swing

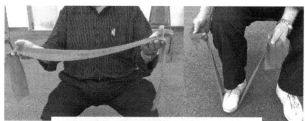

- Scoot to the right edge of the seat, bend forward and put left arm on left knee
- Exhale as you swing right arm forward.  Pause.
- Swing arm backward.  Pause.
- Swing arm forward.  Front to back to front is one repetition.
- Repeat 10-15 times each arm. (optional: dumbbell or can of soup)

# Arms:  Form, Form, Form

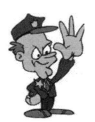

The elbows are just hinges for these exercises.

Whether you're exercising the muscles in the front or the back of the arm, the elbow should stay close to the body and/or stationary throughout the movements.

## Bicep Curl (front of arm)

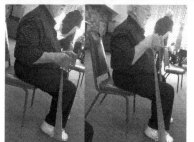

- Grasp ends of band with each hand
- Secure band under foot
- Exhale as you curl fists up toward your shoulders
- Keep elbows tucked into side. Pause.
- **Slowly** lower hands down to start position.
- Repeat 8-15 times

This is where the difficulty of the band tension is important and can easily be adjusted.

You want to go through full range of motion so if the exercise is...
- Too hard?  Slide hands toward end of band
- Too easy?  Slide hands down toward feet

Dumbbell/Cans of Soup.  No, a 12 oz curl (with a bottle of beer) doesn't count!   Hold object in each hand

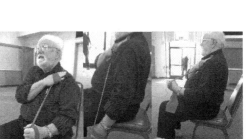

- Tuck elbows into sides
- Curl wrist up toward shoulders
- Squeeze object
- Lower slowly
- Repeat 8-15 times

PROGRESSION:  Try a heavier object.

**Triceps Extension** (back of arm.  Aka, angel wings)

- Band:  Wrap band around palms of hands approximately 10-12 inches apart.
- Pretend to pledge allegiance to the flag as you bring your right hand toward your left shoulder.
- Tuck left elbow into side and bend at forearm in front of body.
- Stand tall, exhale and extend left arm down toward left hip.
- Pause then slowly return left hand to start.
- Keep elbow tucked into side, it is just a hinge

---

**Resistance Band Guidelines**

Do not allow slack in band.

Use slow controlled movements; you are in control of the band.

---

Dumbbell/cans of soup:

- Holding can of soup, right arm is extended is toward ceiling
- Bending at elbow, reach back as if to scratch your back with right hand.  Pause.
- Extend right hand toward ceiling
- Elbow is just a hinge. Keep elbow pointed toward ceiling throughout movement.
- Repeat 10-15 times right hand then repeat with left hand

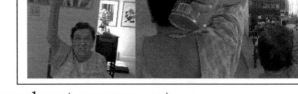

## Abdominals

### Tighten the stomach - PROTECT THE BACK

**Osteoporosis warning**

The stomach muscles are important to help protect your lower back. Tighten the front and protect the back.

If you have severe case of osteoporosis, you want to check with your doctor before doing this exercise

Stomach crunch, with or without band:

- Scoot to the back of your chair with both feet on the floor.
- Cross arms on chest.
- Tighten stomach muscles and exhale as you bend forward. You want to bend over your belly button and feel your elbows tap the top of your thighs.
- Inhale as you return to upright seated position
- Repeat 15-20 times.

Challenge:   Put band around back of chair around armpit level. Cross arms on chest as if crossing your heart.  Tighten band by grabbing back further on band.  Same sequence:

- Tighten stomach; exhale as you curl your shoulders down toward your lap.
- Pretend to curl over your belly button.

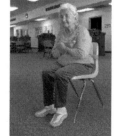

- Pause, squeeze stomach muscles, inhale and return to upright position.

## Back

## PROTECT THE BACK...TIGHTEN THE BELLY!

<u>Elbows back:</u>

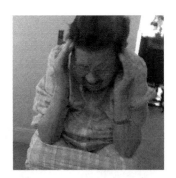

- Sit tall, interlace fingers behind head, elbows out to sides
- Keep upper body straight as you drop chin to chest, rounding forward as you bring elbows together in front.  Tap top of thighs if you can
- Tighten stomach as you lift chest
- Push elbows out to side as you straighten up, lifting chest upward toward the ceiling
- Repeat 5-10 times.

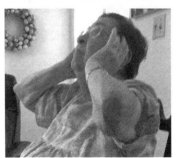

## ALWAYS TIGHTEN STOMACH BEFORE RETURNING TO START

## FLEXIBILITY TRAINING

Defined as the ability to move joints through the full range of motion.

In other words, the ability to move in the way God intended us to move. We need to stretch muscles daily!

## Basic 5 Stretches:

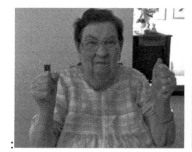 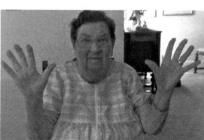

1. <u>Take 5 Hand Squeeze</u>

- Tighten hands into a fist and squeeze
- Then open fingers as wide as possible.
- Tighten, squeeze.
- Repeat 10-15 times.

2. <u>Three (3) circles</u>

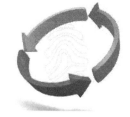

a. Wrist: keep arms still.

- Start moving hands in circular motion
- Keep arm still. Do 10-15 full circles
- Pause and repeat in opposite direction.

b. <u>Arm</u>: keep arms straight.

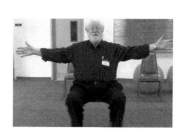

- Extend arms out to side. Thumbs up.
- Start making small circles with arms. Keep arms straight and shoulders down.
- Slowly make bigger circles. Do 10-15 then pause, and repeat in opposite direction.
- Start small then slowly get circles bigger, pretend you are doing the back stroke in a swimming pool

c. <u>Ankle:</u> keep leg still.

- Extend right leg in front of body
- Keep leg still as your draw circles with your toes
- Draw 10-15 circles with toes, big circles.
- Pause and repeat in opposite direction.
- Put foot down and repeat with left foot.

3. <u>Leg extension:</u>  This is to warm up the muscles in your thigh.

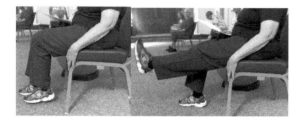

Leg Extension

- Sit tall in the middle of your chair.
- Extend right foot in front of your body.
- Pause, squeeze thigh muscle and return foot toward floor.
- Repeat 10-20 times right leg.  Then do with left leg.
- Do not touch foot to floor.  Squeeze thigh muscle to extend leg, squeeze/pause, lower toward floor

4. <u>Hamstring stretch + knee press</u>

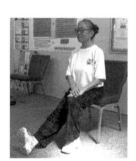

Scoot to edge of seat

- Scoot to edge of seat.
- Extend right in front of you, press heel into floor and extend toes toward the ceiling.

- Knee press: Tighten thigh muscles and try to straighten your right leg.  I call this a knee press b/c you are trying to press the knee down toward the floor.

- <u>DO NOT USE YOUR HANDS TO STRAIGHTEN THE LEG,</u> just tighten thigh muscle to get leg straight.
- Repeat tightening thigh muscle to straighten leg 3 times.

- Sitting tall, stack both hands on bent knee.

- Exhale as you bend forward from the hip.  Keep upper body straight as you shift weight to front of your seat.  Feel stretch in the back of your right leg.  Hold that position.

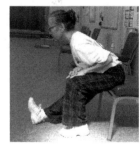

- Then do a knee press (tighten right thigh muscle as if pressing right knee toward floor).  Exhale as you lean further into this stretch.  Be careful, this is a deep stretch.  Hold 10 seconds.

- Relax leg muscle then inhale and exhale as you go for the gusto and <u>try to grab your toes</u>.  Keep upper body straight.  This is a deep stretch, do not bounce.

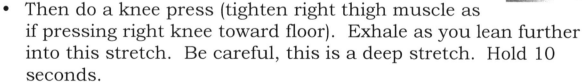

Try to touch toes

- Hold 10-20 seconds. Tighten stomach and come up one vertebrae at a time.

## 5. Kegal squeeze

Incontinence is a common problem among older adults and often results in pre-mature institutionalization.

Do this exercise to strengthen the lower pelvic floor muscles to better control leakage and to avoid embarrassing moments.

And men, this exercise is not for women only! You have pelvic floor muscles, too!

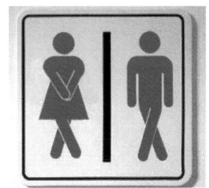

Imagine you are cutting off the flow of urine as you tighten bladder muscles

- Hold for 10 seconds. Release.
- Repeat 10 times.
- Do 2-3 times per day.

## Head to Toe Flexibility

### Neck

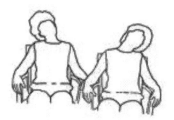

### Neck tilt:

- Sit tall, lift your chest and drop your shoulders.
- Drop your right ear to your right shoulder.
- Using your right hand, reach up and gently pull head toward right shoulder
- Hold as you exhale and release hand pressure
- Inhale as you drag chin across chest and put left ear on left shoulder.
- Reach up with left hand and gently pull head toward left shoulder.
- Exhale then drag chin across chest and tilt head to right
- Repeat 5 times.

## Shoulders

### Shoulder Stretch:

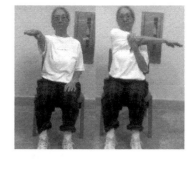

- Extend right arm in front of your body at chest height.
- Bring right arm across your body and with left hand, push right elbow closer toward body.
- Enjoy the stretch in your right shoulder.
- Hold for 10 seconds then do with the left arm.

## CHEST

### Tight chest+ Loose back muscles= Poor posture.

### Chest stretch:

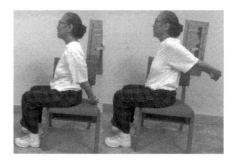

- Clasp hands behind body.
- Sit tall with shoulders over hips, tighten belly and exhale as you raise straight arms as high as you can behind you.
- Keep upper body braced and straight and try not to lean too far forward as raise extended arms behind you.
- Relax.  Repeat 5 times.

### Wrists

### Fingers Up, Fingers Down:

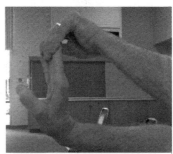

- Extend right arm in front of body, fingers up toward the ceiling.
- With left hand, pull fingertips of right hand back toward body.
- Feel stretch in bottom of forearm
- Drop fingers to face the floor
- With left hand, grab fingers and pull back toward body, pushing wrist forward.  Feel stretch in top of wrist
- Hold 5-10 seconds, then repeat with left hand.

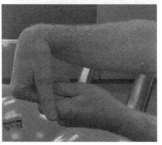

### Triceps

### Pat yourself on the back:

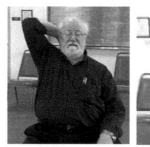
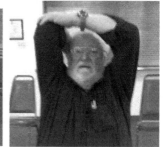

- Extend right arm overhead.
- Bend right arm at elbow to pat yourself on the back.
- Grab right elbow with left hand and gently pull right elbow toward your head.
- Lean to the right into the stretch.
- Repeat with left hand.

### Back

### Mat cat/Mellow cat:

- Scoot yourself to the back of your chair Sitting tall in homebase with feet on the floor
- Press lower back into back of chair. You can round forward at the shoulders to resemble a "mad" cat.
- Stretch then return to neutral (homebase).
- Exhale as you arch back off the back of the chair, rotating arms backward, lifting chest like a "Happy" cat.
- Return to neutral.  Repeat 3-8 times.

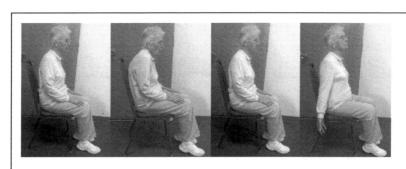

Neutral    Mad Cat    Neutral    Mellow Cat

## Thighs

### Standing next to chair:

- Bend right knee behind you and grab right ankle with left hand
- Squeeze right thigh muscle then relax. Hold 20-30 seconds.
- Put foot down and repeat with left leg.

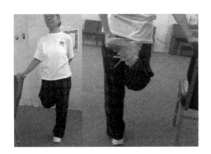

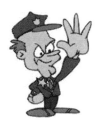

This cross over will help you keep your spine straight as you do this stretch.

Keep knee facing the floor as you squeeze and tighten the thigh muscle.

### Lying on side quad stretch:

- Lay on left side. Bend right knee behind body as if doing a butt kicker.
- Grab right ankle with right hand. Keep knee pointing toward feet. Squeeze thigh muscle, hold 10-20 seconds
- Roll to other side and repeat with left leg.

***If you cannot reach your ankle, use a towel or resistance band around foot and gently pull back toward body***

## Inner thigh

### Straddle stretch behind chair:

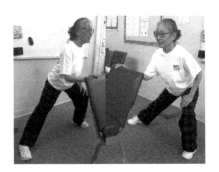

- Stand behind chair with legs as wide apart as comfortable with hands on chair and chest upright.
- Exhale as you shift weight to right foot.
- Slide hips over and butt goes back as if to tap wall. Left leg is straight. Feel the stretch in inner left thigh. Push butt back toward wall and keep body straight.

- Return to center.
- Exhale as you shift weight to leftside, bending left knee as you accept weight onto LEFT foot. Keep right leg straight. Left butt goes back toward wall. EXHALE. Hold 10-15 seconds.
- Repeat 3-5 times in each direction. Hold stretch and lean upper body to feel stretch.

---

**Million Dollar Tip:**

Momma always told you not to stick your butt out but she was wrong for this stretch! The further you stick your butt back and straighter you keep your leg, the deeper the stretch!

**Stick it out!**

---

## Hips

### "This stretch is a real pain in the butt"...

- Seated tall, lift right foot up and place on top of left knee.

- Keep back straight as you bend forward from the hips, gently pressing down on your right knee.

- Relax as this is an intense stretch in your right hip/butt area.

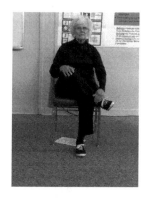

- Hold stretch for 15-30 seconds, hinge forward from hip to increase stretch

- Repeat on the left side

## Hamstrings

## Standing hamstring stretch:

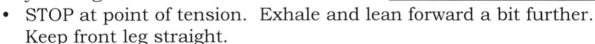
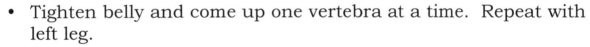

- Stand behind a chair and extend right foot in front of body with heel on ground, toes toward ceiling.
- Shift weight to back foot as you hinge forward from hip. *Keep upper body straight.* Hold onto chair to support upper body weight and back.
- Reach forward toward toes with opposite hand, pushing hips back as you hinge forward.
- STOP at point of tension. Exhale and lean forward a bit further. Keep front leg straight.
- Tighten belly and come up one vertebra at a time. Repeat with left leg.

REMINDER: This is NOT a balance exercise but a stretch! Hold onto the chair or place hand on left thigh for support. Hold stretch for 15-30 seconds.

Or stay seated....

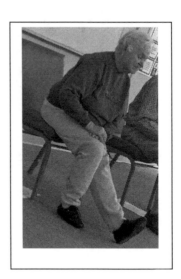

## ENDURANCE EXERCISES

Anything you enjoy that involves total body activity.

Think VERBS:

**Walking**          **Bicycling**          **Boating**

**Housecleaning**    **Gardening**          **Dancing**

**Hiking**           **Vacuuming**

**Washing the car**

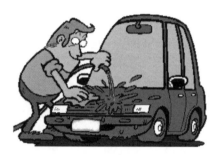

Although we may consider some of these as endurance activities,

**<u>The Following List Will Not Bring The Fall Prevention Benefits I Am Talking About:</u>**

Running errands            Resting

Knitting                   Reading

Sleeping                   Napping

Eating                     Taking a break

Daydreaming                Watching someone else exercise

# Walking

One of the best forms of cardiovascular exercise, walking doesn't cost you a dime and can be done anywhere.  If you can't walk, you can probably march in your chair.

Whether you march in place from your wheelchair or speed walk around the park, we have a **built-in balance mechanism** that God equipped each of us with.

The built-in components are our arms and legs and the balance mechanism is picking up opposite arm and opposite leg while walking.

If you have ever attended one of my educational, interactive workshops, you have tried this and probably struggled getting started. This is not as easy as you might think, especially if you have been using a walker or a cane for a long time.

### Opposite arm, opposite leg:

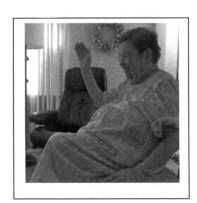

- Pick up the left foot as you bend the right arm.
- Keep your trunk still, shoulders relaxed.
- Swing the arms only.

Due to weakness in legs and hips, it may be difficult to shift weight to one side and truly 'pick up' your feet as you march in place.

Try this seated.

- Pretend you have a string attaching the left knee and the right fist.  Every time you bend your wrist upward, the opposite knee comes up.
- Practice lifting left knee and right fist 10 times.
- Repeat with right knee and left fist

Practice alternating right knee then left knee, trying to bend opposite arm with each knee lift.

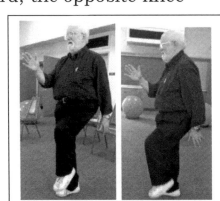

Seated marching:

Lift knees DIFFERENT HEIGHTS:

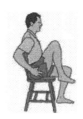

- LOW
- MEDIUM
- HIGH

Swing arms by side: OPPOSITE ARM with OPPOSITE LEG!

Now stand up in front of a wall and behind your chair. I'm serious...this opposite arm/opposite leg thing can be tricky!

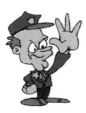

Keep your chin parallel to the floor, chest lifted and eyes focused on a vertical target.

And drop those shoulders!

## MILLION DOLLAR TIP: DROP YOUR SHOULDERS

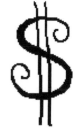

The reason I continually cue about dropping those shoulders is because we carry so much of life's tension in our neck and upper back muscles.

When we become fearful, we tense up. That tension builds up in our muscles. Unaware of our posture, our shoulders are naturally pulled upward toward the neck.

Think about walking heel to toe, without holding onto the wall or counter. With your eyes closed. If you become fearful, your shoulders are probably connected to your ears just thinking about that situation!

Now stop and relax. Drop your shoulders. Consciously think about tucking your shoulder blades into your back pockets as you lift up from your chest. Wow...what a difference, huh?

The message I want to get across about the shoulders is that tension is subconscious. **Fear triggers tension.** You have to constantly think about your posture and dropping your shoulders, especially while doing balance challenges that push you out of your comfort zone!

# Walking Gait Training

The goal is develop a flexible and adaptable gait pattern so you are better able to cross street different speeds, maneuver in and out of crowds and respond to changes in environment in an efficient manner. For instance, you many need to make sudden stops and starts, avoid obstacles, and alter walking gait patterns to avoid collisions and near falls.

The ability to think on the fly can determine if you lose your balance or if you are able to avoid a potentially hazardous situation. There are several different walking patterns that I have my clients practice.

I have them practice walking these patterns and in class I will call out a number and have them respond. Try having a friend or loved one call out 1, 2, 3, or 4 and see if you can:

1) Remember the walking gait

2) Do it!

This is how we train the body to do what the brain tells it to. Quickly. On the fly.

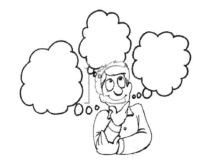

 Gait patterns:

**#1-Narrow:** Walk as if you are walking a plank. Not necessarily heel to toe but this gait is more narrow than you are used to walking. You will probably feel a little unsteady at first so practice this walking gait near a wall or counter.

**#2-Wide:** Waddle, waddle. Get those feet wide and take big steps. This stride will be easier since the walking gait naturally gets wider as we age because we don't like to stand on one leg too long. I've heard everything from 'this is like walking with a dirty diaper' to "I feel like a duck".

**#3-Tip Toes:** Tip-toe through the tulips....pretend the string on top of your head is pulling you up toward the ceiling as you walk forward. Bring your belly button forward with you! Try not to let the heels come in contact with the floor and yes....DROP YOUR SHOULDERS! You definitely may want to try this next to a wall or kitchen counter at first until your ankles get stronger.

**#4-Heels:** OK, this requires a total shift in direction....lift the toes and walk on the heels only. To adjust to my belly button being back so far, I stick my butt back and bring my chest slightly forward. That helps me balance and walk on my heels so stick your butt back and ever so slightly lean forward as you keep your toes from touching the floor.

Try practicing each of these walking patterns. If you cannot walk, do them seated. The placement of the feet is our base of support. Keeping our belly button over the feet is the goal to balance.

**#5-Wedding March:** It may have been years ago, you may have never done it or if you're like me, you've practiced this a couple of times! This walking gait is exactly like the wedding march down the aisle. You take a long stride with right foot, step up to homebase, then take a long stride with left foot, step up to homebase.

To begin, I want you to step forward with right foot only. The bigger your stride, the more difficult it will be so start with short steps. Walk across the room leading with right foot only, pause as you bring left foot forward to homebase. Keep upper body tall and eyes focused on vertical target.

Repeat leading with left foot only. Then alternate right and left foot. Remember to start with small steps and take longer strides as you get stronger.

> *As we walk through life, there are changes in our environment that require us to take the narrow path, maybe straddle the creek at times, or we may have to quietly tip-toe past trouble and I know there are times when we have to dig our heels in and just march forward so do each one of these walking patterns while keeping your chin up, eyes focused on a vertical target, chest lifted and by God, where are your shoulders? They are down!*

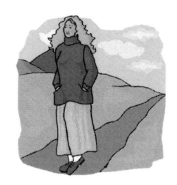

## Stop Wide

Ok. Balance is about keeping the belly button over the feet. When you walk, you may have to make sudden stops. I recommend stopping with a wide stance to maintain better balance.

Suppose it's Christmas, the mall is crowded and you are window shopping. Something catches your eye in the window so you stop to get a better look when suddenly, a young kid comes barreling around the corner and bumps into you.

Scenario 1: When you stopped, you stood there as you always do, not paying attention to your posture and your feet are probably close together. You have a narrow 'base of support'.

Scenario 2: You listened to the Fall Prevention Lady's advice and stopped wide. Your feet are at least hip-width apart, your knees are slightly bent and you are ready for anything!

Quickly recall the earlier balance training segment where you stood with your toes and heels together. You felt a lot less stable with your feet together than you did with feet hip-width apart.

Now think about the walking patterns. It's a lot easier to do walking pattern #2 (wide) than it is to do walking pattern #1 (narrow). The moral of the story is to **stop with your feet wide.**

### FEET WIDE WHEN YOU STOP

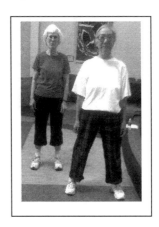

You are much less likely to lose your balance when your feet are in a wide stance than when you are standing with feet together or one foot in front of the other. This will be especially helpful out in crowds and during holiday seasons.

- Make a conscious effort
- Make it obvious for all to see

**GREAT ENDURANCE BUILDER!!!**

**Marching with head turns:**

- Marching in place behind chair
- March for 8 counts, turn head to right.
- March for 8 counts then turn head to center.
- March 8 counts. Turn head to left.
- Then try marching without stopping head at center (just look from right to left).
- March 6 counts, turn head to right.
- March 6 steps, turn head to left.
- Repeat 20-30 seconds at a time

**Progressions:**

- Lower count to 4 steps before turning head.
- Change marching patterns. Try #1, 2, 3 and 4 while doing head turns.
- March in place then start walking patterns with head turns.

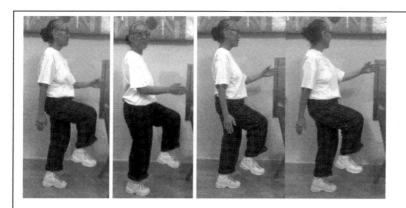

**LOOK FOR A VERTICAL TARGET EACH TIME YOU TURN YOUR HEAD!!!**

## Cool Down

Breathe deeply to bring heart rate back to resting level. It's always good to relax and do some gentle stretches at the end of exercise session.

Here's a light stretching routine I have my classes do after Balance Training 101™.

- Shoulder shrugs
- Shoulder rolls
- Chest stretch
- Hamstring stretch
- Calf stretch

**Breath deep.** Congratulate yourself for making the time to do this exercise routine today and taking responsibility for your well-being by reducing the risk of a fall.

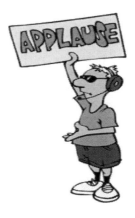

# Great Job!!!

## PART III: FACILITATE

## All This Information...Now What?

I have given you a lot information about falls and how to reduce the risk of an accidental fall. Now what are you supposed to do with it?

1. Start at home with the home safety checklist. Go through each room in the house and look for potentially hazardous situations.

- Pick up throw rugs or put double-sided adhesive tape on back
- Remove clutter
- Put in night lights

2. Start exercising at home. I just gave you 30 pages of exercises but all I'm asking is that you start with at least 10 minutes a day.

Recall there are four different types of exercise you should be doing to improve your balance and prevent falls. I created charts to monitor your progress and to make it easy for you to follow a well-balanced fall prevention exercise program at home. Use what you need.

For anyone who downloaded this from the computer, just print the page with the chart and post somewhere visible!

The list of charts is on the following page, followed by the charts and then the Index.

## List of Charts

1.  Balance Training 101™:  4 weeks of progressively challenging balance training exercise routines and weekly balance adherence checklists.  Try to practice these exercises at least three times a week.

2.  Strength-building:  List of exercises for entire body.  Try to do at least twice a week.

3.  Flexibility and Postural Awareness:  Basic 5 stretches and Postural Awareness activities to be done daily.  List of "Head to Toe" flexibility activities to be done at your leisure when you have the time.

4.  Week-at-a-Glance:  checklist of the different types of exercises you should be doing each week to prevent falls.  Post on your refrigerator or someplace you will see everyday!

5.  Daily Stretch Checklist: includes the Basic 5 stretches, postural awareness exercises and simple lower body strengthening exercises.


## Balance Training 101™

As you learned, balance is about muscles and senses and keeping your belly button over your feet.  I want you to train your muscles at least twice a week and your senses at least three times a week.

When you train your balance using this program, you will do at least two (2) exercises.

You will train ONE of your senses (Using the "It Makes Sense" exercises) and pair that with either a Belly button activity or Walking Gait exercise.

Got it?  Here it is again in words...


## How to train your balance.

Pick an exercise that targets your eyes, your ears, or your feet ("It Makes Sense" training).  That's one exercise.  Then you will choose either a BELLY BUTTON OR WALKING GAIT exercise.

These exercises should be individualized to your ability and as you improve, increase the challenge of the exercise with different progressions.

Balance Descriptive

I created four weeks of balance training routines and there are new exercises each week that are noted by an asterisk.

I call these charts the "Balance Descriptive". See sample for Week 1:

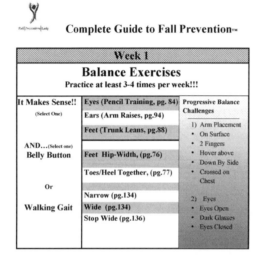

Balance Checklist

I also provide four weekly checklists to monitor your balance training. This is a chart to check off the weekly balance exercises that are listed on the balance descriptive. Print (or make copies if you have the book) and post so you can check off exercises as you do them.

See sample balance training checklist for Week 1 below:

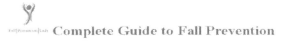

Complete Guide to Fall Prevention

# Weekly CheckList Week 1

| CheckOff List | MON | TUE | WED | THU | FRI | SAT | SUN |
|---|---|---|---|---|---|---|---|
| **Balance** | | | | | | | |
| It Makes Sense | | | | | | | |
| Eyes | | | | | | | |
| Ears | | | | | | | |
| Feet | | | | | | | |
| Belly Button | | | | | | | |
| Feet Hip Width | | | | | | | |
| Toe/Heel Together | | | | | | | |
| Walking | | | | | | | |
| Narrow | | | | | | | |
| Wide | | | | | | | |

Do NOT try exercise progressions until you are ready!

## Progressions

- DO NOT PROGRESS to more challenging exercise unless you are confident and feel ready.

- There's a huge difference between holding onto a surface and putting your arms down by your sides so I created two surface progressions:
    - o 2 fingers: Hold onto surface with only 2 fingers
    - o Hover above: Try to hover your hands above the surface while you practice

- TRY to do a progression. Change your arm placement. Alter the position of your feet. Try to close your eyes.

Remember, not everyone responds the same and not everyone will progress at the same rate.

### Take your time and stick with it!

OK, so that's the balance part. At least three times a week, I want you to do an "It Makes Sense" exercise AND a Belly Button OR Walking Gait exercise.

You choose but don't always do the same exercises. If you have questions about a specific exercise, contact me with questions. info@thefallpreventionlady.com

4 weeks of Weekly balance exercise descriptions and Weekly balance check-off lists are next.

Print these out and follow along each week.

## 4 Weekly Balance Descriptives and Checklists

### Week 1: Balance Descriptive

Fall|Prevention|Lady

# Complete Guide to Fall Prevention™

| Week 1 | | |
|---|---|---|
| **Balance Exercises** Practice at least 3-4 times per week!!! | | |
| **It Makes Sense!!** (Select One) | Eyes (Pencil Training, pg. 85) | **Progressive Balance Challenges** |
| | Ears (Arm Raises, pg.95) | 1) Arm Placement |
| | Feet (Trunk Leans, pg.89) | • On Surface |
| **AND...**(Select one) **Belly Button** | Feet Hip-Width, (pg.77) | • 2 Fingers • Hover above • Down By Side |
| | Toes/Heel Together, (pg.78) | • Crossed on Chest |
| Or | Narrow (pg.131) | 2) Eyes |
| **Walking Gait** | Wide (pg.131) | • Eyes Open |
| | Stop Wide (pg.133) | • Dark Glasses • Eyes Closed |

## Week 1: Balance Checklist

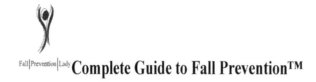

Fall|Prevention|Lady **Complete Guide to Fall Prevention™**

# Week 1 Balance CheckList

**Practice 3-4 times each week!!**

| CheckOff List | MON | TUE | WED | THU | FRI | SAT | SUN |
|---|---|---|---|---|---|---|---|
| **Balance** | | | | | | | |
| It Makes Sense | | | | | | | |
| Eyes | | | | | | | |
| Ears | | | | | | | |
| Feet | | | | | | | |
| Belly Button | | | | | | | |
| Feet Hip Width | | | | | | | |
| Toe/Heel Together | | | | | | | |
| Walking | | | | | | | |
| Narrow | | | | | | | |
| Wide | | | | | | | |

Do NOT try exercise progressions until you are ready!

## Week 2:  Balance Descriptive

Fall|Prevention|Lady

# Complete Guide to Fall Prevention™

| Week 2 |
|---|
| **Balance Exercises**<br>Practice at least 3-4 times per week !!! |

| It Makes Sense!!<br>(Select One)<br><br><br><br>AND...<br>(Select one)<br><br>Belly Button<br><br>Or<br><br>Walking Gait | Eyes (Pencil Training, pg. 85)<br>Ears (Arm Raises, pg.95)<br>Feet (Trunk Leans, pg.89)<br><br>Feet  Hip-Width,  (pg.77)<br>Toe/Heel Together,  (pg.78)<br>*Split  Stance,  (pg.78)<br><br>Narrow, (pg.131)<br>Wide, (pg.131)<br>*Tip Toes, (pg.131) | Progressive Balance Challenges<br>———<br>1) Arm Placement<br>• On Surface<br>• 2 Fingers<br>• Hover above<br>• Down By Side<br>Crossed on<br>Chest<br><br>2)  Eyes<br>• Eyes Open<br>• Dark Glasses<br>• Eyes Closed |

*New Exercise for this week

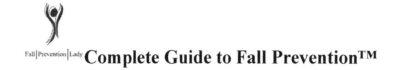

**Complete Guide to Fall Prevention™**

# Week 2 Balance CheckList

## Practice 3-4 times each week!!

| CheckOff List | MON | TUE | WED | THU | FRI | SAT | SUN |
|---|---|---|---|---|---|---|---|
| **Balance** | | | | | | | |
| **It Makes Sense** | | | | | | | |
| Eyes | | | | | | | |
| Ears | | | | | | | |
| Feet | | | | | | | |
| Belly Button | | | | | | | |
| Feet  Hip Width | | | | | | | |
| Toe/Heel Together | | | | | | | |
| *Split  Stance | | | | | | | |
| Walking | | | | | | | |
| Narrow | | | | | | | |
| Wide | | | | | | | |
| *Tip Toes | | | | | | | |

*New Exercise!!

Do NOT try exercise progressions until you are ready!

## Week 3: Balance Descriptive

Fall|Prevention|Lady

# Complete Guide to Fall Prevention™

| Week 3 | | |
|---|---|---|
| **Balance Exercises** Practice at least 3-4 times Per Week !!!! | | |
| **It Makes Sense!!** (Select One) | **Eyes** (Seated or Standing) **Pencil Training (pg.85)** **Ears** Arm Raises (pg.95) *March in Place w/Head turns (pg.97, 134) **Feet** **Trunk Leans (pg.89)** | Progressive Balance Challenges _____ 1) Arm Placement • On Surface • 2 Fingers • Hover above • Down By Side • Crossed on Chest |
| **AND...** (Select one) **Belly Button** **Or** **Walking Gait** | Feet Hip-Width (pg.77) Toe/Heel Together (pg.78) Split Stance (pg.78) Narrow (pg.131) Wide (pg.131) Tip Toes (pg.131) *Heels (pg.132) | 2) Eyes • Eyes Open • Dark Glasses • Eyes Closed 3) Feet • Wide • Together • Split Stance |
| **Reaction Strategy** | *Ankle Leans (pg.98) | |

*New Exercise this Week

## Week 3:  Balance Checklist

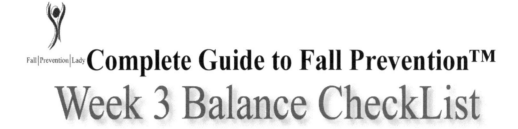

**Complete Guide to Fall Prevention™**

# Week 3 Balance CheckList

## Practice 3-4 times each week!!

| CheckOff List | MON | TUE | WED | THU | FRI | SAT | SUN |
|---|---|---|---|---|---|---|---|
| **Balance** | | | | | | | |
| **It Makes Sense** | | | | | | | |
| Eyes | | | | | | | |
| Ears | | | | | | | |
| Feet | | | | | | | |
| Belly Button | | | | | | | |
| Feet  Hip Width | | | | | | | |
| Toe/Heel Together | | | | | | | |
| Split  Stance | | | | | | | |
| Walking | | | | | | | |
| Narrow | | | | | | | |
| Wide | | | | | | | |
| Tip Toes | | | | | | | |
| *Heels | | | | | | | |
| Reaction Strategy | | | | | | | |
| *Ankle Leans | | | | | | | |

*New Exercise!!

Do NOT try exercise progressions until you are ready!

## Week 4: Balance Descriptive

Fall|Prevention|Lady

# Complete Guide to Fall Prevention™

| Week 4 Balance Exercises Practice at least 3-4 times per Week!!! | | |
|---|---|---|
| **It Makes Sense!!**<br>(Select One) | **Eyes** (Seated or Standing) | Progressive Balance Challenges |
| | **Pencil Training (pg.85)** | |
| | **Ears** | |
| | **Arm Raises (pg.95)** | 1) Arm Placement |
| | **March in place w/Headturns (pg.97, 134)** | • On Surface |
| | | • 2 Fingers |
| | **Feet** | • Hover above |
| | **Trunk Leans (pg.89)** | • Down By Side |
| **AND...** | **Feet Hip-Width (pg.77)** | • Crossed on Chest |
| (Select one) | **Toe/Heel Together (pg.78)** | |
| **Belly Button** | **Split Stance (pg.78)** | 2) Eyes |
| | ***Semi-Tandem (pg.81)** | |
| | **Narrow (pg.131)** | • Eyes Open |
| **Or** | **Wide (pg.131)** | • Dark Glasses |
| **Walking Gait** | **Tip Toes (pg.131)** | • Eyes Closed |
| | **Heels (pg.132)** | 3) Feet |
| | ***Wedding March! (pg.132)** | • Wide |
| | | • Together |
| | | • Split Stance |
| **Reaction Strategy** | **Ankle Leans (pg.98)** | |

*New Exercise this Week

## Week 4:  Balance Checklist

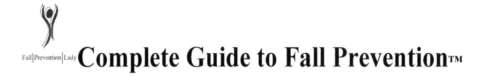

**Complete Guide to Fall Prevention™**

## Week 4 Balance CheckList

### Practice 3-4 times each week!!

| CheckOff List | MON | TUE | WED | THU | FRI | SAT | SUN |
|---|---|---|---|---|---|---|---|
| **Balance** | | | | | | | |
| **It Makes Sense** | | | | | | | |
| Eyes | | | | | | | |
| Ears | | | | | | | |
| Feet | | | | | | | |
| Belly Button | | | | | | | |
| Feet  Hip Width | | | | | | | |
| Toe/Heel Together | | | | | | | |
| Split  Stance | | | | | | | |
| *Tandem | | | | | | | |
| Walking | | | | | | | |
| Narrow | | | | | | | |
| Wide | | | | | | | |
| Tip Toes | | | | | | | |
| Heels | | | | | | | |
| *Wedding March | | | | | | | |
| Reaction Strategy | | | | | | | |
| Ankle Leans | | | | | | | |

*New Exercise!!

Do NOT try exercise progressions until you are ready!

## Strengthening Exercises

Staying strong is the number one way to prevent falls.

Twice a week, I want you to go through a total body strengthening program.

In other words, I want you to do one exercise for each major body part (Hips, Legs, Back, Chest, Shoulders, Arms, Stomach).

Try to do 8-15 repetitions of each exercise.

**A list of strengthening exercises is on the following page.**

If you forget how to do an exercise, I listed the page number that describes the exercise to refresh your memory.

Remember, you must **keep those legs strong!**

- Do your toe and heel lifts
- Point and flex your toes
- Keep drawing ankle circles
- Kick your heel to the wall
- Chair stands, chair stands, chair stands

Strengthening exercise routine to follow....

## Strengthening Exercises

 **Complete Guide to Fall Prevention™**

| Strength |
|---|
| Exercise at least 2 times per week --One Exercise per Body Part |

**Hips**
- Clam (pg.105)
- Foot to Wall (pg.105)

**Legs**
- Chair Stand (pg.107)
- Front & Rear Leg Lifts (pg.111)

**Calves/Ankles**
- Toe Raises/Heel Raises (pg.110-111)
- Point Flex (pg.111)

**Back**
- Seated Row (pg.113)
- 1 Arm Row (pg. 113)

**Chest**
- Press (pg.114)
- Stretch (pg.114)

**Shoulders**
- Horizontal Pull (pg.115)
- Open Refrigerator Door (pg.115)

**Bicep**
- Curl (Band or Weight) (pg.116 or 117)

**Triceps**
- Elbow Extension (Band or Weight) (pg.117 or 118)

**Abs (Seated)**
- Stomach Crunch (pg.118)

**Back**
- Elbows Back (pg.119)

**Do 8-15 repetitions per exercise and don't forget to breathe!**

## Flexibility and Postural Awareness Activities

*"You must stretch what you strengthen*

*and strengthen what you stretch"*

~ K. Ward

Stretching is important to keep your muscles, tendons, ligaments and connective tissue moving as they should, especially when you are doing your strengthening exercises.

### Stretching also helps to reduce stress.

It's a great idea if you can make stretching part of your daily routine. Find a time that works for you and take 5 minutes to do some stretches. Breathe deep. Relax. Hold each stretch at least 30 seconds.

## And don't bounce!

I have included the <u>Basic 5 Stretches</u> (included on all of my Take 5 to Exercise seated stretching and strengthening DVDs).

These Basic 5 Stretches can be done anywhere, anytime.

For days when you have more time to stretch and relax, I have included the <u>"Head to Toe" stretches</u>. Once you start stretching, the "feel good" juices will start to flow and you will want to do more.

As I mentioned in the Guide, one way to improve your balance is to be more aware of your posture.

That's why I have included <u>Postural Awareness Exercises</u> along with Flexibility so you are more aware of your posture every day.

## Basic 5 Stretches and Postural Awareness Activities

Fall|Prevention|Lady

# Complete Guide to Fall Prevention
# Flexibility
### DAILY    Create Your Own 10 minute Routine!!

## Basic 5 Stretches

1. **Take 5 Hand Squeeze** (pg.120)
2. **Three Circles** (pg.120)
   - **Wrist**
   - **Arm**
   - **Ankle**
3. **Leg Extension** (pg.121)
4. **Hamstring Stretch** (pg.121)
5. **Kegal Squeeze** (pg.122)

## Posture Exercises

- Seated and Standing Postural Checklist (pg.73)
- Check your window (pg. 76)
- Tighten and Hold (pg.74)

### Posture Progressions
1. Eyes
   - Eyes Open
   - Eyes Closed

2. Arm Placement
   - On Surface
   - 2 Fingers
   - Hover above
   - Down By Side
   - Crossed on Chest

3. Feet
   - Wide
   - Together

## Head to Toe Flexibility:

 **Complete Guide to Fall Prevention™**

| Head to Toe Flexibility |
|---|
| One Exercise per Body Part |

**Neck**
- Neck Tilt (pg.122)

**Shoulders**
- Shoulder Stretch (pg.123)

**Chest**
- Seated Chest Stretch (pg.123)

**Wrists**
- Fingers Up, Fingers Down (pg.123)

**Triceps**
- Pat Yourself on the Back (pg.124)

**Back**
- Mad Cat/Mellow Cat (pg.124)

**Thighs**
- Standing (pg.125)
- Lying (pg.125)
- Inner Thigh Stretch (pg. 125)

**Hips**
- This is a Pain in the Butt! (pg.126)

**Hamstrings**
- Standing (pg.127)
- Seated (pg.127)

**Hold stretches at least 15 seconds and do not bounce!**

Ok, there are **four different types** of exercise to prevent falls:

1. Balance training 101™ should be done at least three times a week. You pick eyes, ears or feet and combine that training with belly button or walking gait exercises.

2. Strength building exercises should be done at least twice a week. Total body exercises are on page 150.

3. Flexibility and postural awareness activities should be done daily. The Basic 5 stretches are quick and can be done anywhere. And don't forget to check your window. When you have time, try to stretch from "Head to Toe"!

The fourth type of exercise in your fall prevention exercise program is endurance. If you are doing the other 3 types of exercise in addition to daily chores, you are also building your endurance!

Try to do something active each day. March in place, walk around the block, vacuum the rug, wash the car, take the dog for a walk, go for a bike ride. Do something to get your body moving.

### "Week-At-A-Glance"

I know this is a lot to remember so I made the "Week-at-a-Glance" adherence chart for you to follow.

**Post this on your refrigerator (or someplace visible)**. Check off the exercises as you do them.

- This DOES NOT HAVE to be overwhelming.
- Take 10 minutes a day and do what you can.
- Designate certain days to balance and some days to strengthening.
- Everyday do some stretching and be aware of your posture.

As you get familiar with the exercises, this will be easy!

Fall│Prevention│Lady **Complete Guide to Fall Prevention**

# Week At A Glance

## Fall Prevention Exercise Program

**Week At A Glance**

| Weekly Overview | MON | TUE | WED | THU | FRI | SAT | SUN |
|---|---|---|---|---|---|---|---|
| **Balance** | | | | | | | |
| It Makes Sense | | | | | | | |
| Eyes | | | | | | | |
| Ears | | | | | | | |
| Feet | | | | | | | |
| Belly Button | | | | | | | |
| Walking Gait | | | | | | | |
| **Strength** | | | | | | | |
| Hips | | | | | | | |
| Legs | | | | | | | |
| Back | | | | | | | |
| Chest | | | | | | | |
| Arms | | | | | | | |
| **Flexibility** | | | | | | | |
| Basic 5 | | | | | | | |
| **Posture** | | | | | | | |
| Check Your Window | | | | | | | |
| Tighten and Hold | | | | | | | |
| **Endurance** | | | | | | | |

# Daily Stretch Checklist

Have you ever used Cliff notes while in school?  If you recall, cliff notes summarize an entire book in about 50 pages.  I've developed a fall prevention version of cliff notes called the "The Fall Prevention Lady's Daily Exercise Checklist.

If you don't do anything else, try to go through this list each day. This list includes the Basic 5 stretches and some postural and strengthening exercises.  It's a great place to start but remember this is your program so design what works for you.

---

**Daily Stretching Checklist**

_____        **Take 5 Hand Squeeze**

**3 Circles**
_____                **Wrist**

_____                **Arm**

_____                **Ankle**

_____        **Leg Extension**

_____        **Hamstring Stretch**

_____        **Kegal Squeeze**

_____        **Practice Postural awareness:  Standing and Seated**

_____        **Check Your Window**

_____        **Toe Lifts**              **Goal number:_____**

_____        **Heel Lifts**             **Goal number:_____**

_____        **Chair Stands**          **Goal number:_____**

_____        **Heel to Wall**          **Goal number:_____**

_____        **Calf Stretch**

**Hold stretches for at least 30 seconds**
**Increase number of chair stands.  Break into 2 sets, if necessary**

**The Fall Prevention Lady**
**Kelly Ward**
**http://www.thefallpreventionlady.com**
**wardkelly@mac.com**
**(916) 821-5715**

---

## INDEX

In the following Index, you will find:

- How To Get Up If You Fall
- Medications That Increase The Risk Of Falls
- Home Safety Checklist
- Senior Resource Directory

I hope you found this Guide to be helpful and that you better understand what is involved in your balance and how you can train your body systems.

Hopefully, you will be able make some changes in your life that will reduce the risk of a fall and keep you independent for as long as possible.

Education is the tool.  Hope is the message.  Change is empowering.

The program works when you work it.

Be safe!  Be patient!  Be consistent!


The Fall Prevention Lady

# Help! I've Fallen and I CAN Get Up!

Falls are accidents and despite our best efforts, accidents happen.

For this reason, I am going to tell you how to get up in case of a fall. Here's what to do:

1. Once on the ground, I want you to forget about whatever you were doing BEFORE the fall. Whatever it was can wait.
2. I want you to take a deep breath. A fall is a traumatic event and you are probably scared. Breathe deep and remain calm.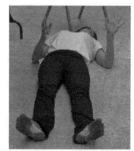
3. Lying on the ground, I want you to wiggle your fingers and toes to make sure everything is ok.
4. If you know something is hurt and have a medical alert system (lifeline), press the button. If not, yell so a neighbor can hear you.

---

This is why it is important to have a medical alert button such as Vital Link or Lifeline if you live alone!

If not, get in the habit of carrying your cell phone with you at all times in case of emergencies.

---

5. Once you feel ok and are ready to get up, I want you to extend one arm overhead and bend the opposite knee.
6. Roll to the side of your body that the arm is extended (the extended arm will protect your neck as you roll) and you will feel your bent knee come in contact with the floor.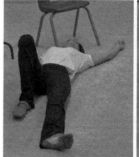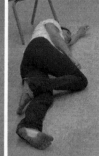
7. From here, push yourself up to your hands and knees.
8. Once on all fours, you can crawl to the couch, chair or bed to pull yourself up.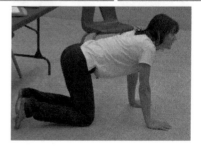

No one said it had to be pretty and I'm sure each one of us has a "unique" way of getting up from the floor so do what you do to get yourself up to the chair, couch or bed safely.

If you are in the middle of the yard, in a parking lot or somewhere **without something to grab onto**, I want you to do the following:

At this point you are on your hands and knees.

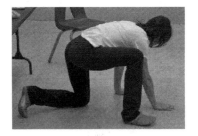

9.   Swing your best leg forward and form a triangle with your hands and the foot of the leg you swung forward.  One hand is the upper part of the triangle while your other hand and the foot will form the base of the triangle.

10. Once you have formed the triangle, I want you to start rocking back and forth to gain some momentum.  The hand that is the upper part of the triangle will stop you from falling forward.

**A body in motion tends to stay in motion so start rocking back and forth to get up!**

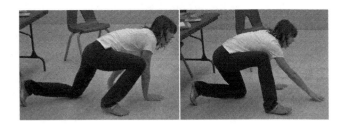

11.Once you have gained enough momentum and are ready to get up, I want you to take a deep breath and swing the other foot forward.

12. From here, you are ready to stand up. SLOWLY. Crawl your hands up your body as you straighten up. Very slowly.

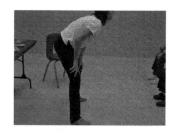

13. Pause when your hands are resting on your knees. And pause again after you begin to straighten up and your hands are on your hips.

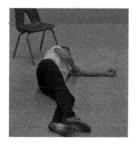

Remember to stand up slowly because we all know what happens when we get up too quickly... you get dizzy and fall down.

## BAD KNEES

If you have bad knees and there is no way you can get onto all fours, here's what I want you to do:

1. Relax. Take a deep breath, whatever you were doing before you fell can wait.
2. Wiggle your fingers and toes. If you are not ok, press your medical alert button or yell for help.
3. If everything is ok, I want you to roll onto your belly.

4. Press your forearms into the floor and begin to walk your hands back toward your body. (I like to keep my entire forearm in contact with the floor because my arm is stronger than my wrist).

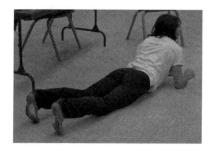

5. As you are walking your hands in toward your body, I want you to imagine that someone is pulling you up by the seat of your pants. In other words, your hips are lifting up toward the ceiling as your hands get closer to body.

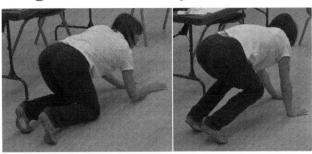

This requires a lot of upper body strength so if you have bad knees, I strongly recommend that you *consistently* work to strengthen the muscles in your arms, chest and shoulders. See strengthening exercises in Part 2 of this book (p.105-121).

## HOW DO I FALL?

A lot of people ask me if there is a "right" way to fall.

The answer is "NO!"

Falls happen so quickly that you probably aren't going to have time to react in a prescribed way. If I tell you to do something and you try to remember and do that as you're falling, you could severely hurt yourself because you didn't do what you could have done in that particular situation.

Some people have heard do not stick your hand out. Well, if you don't stick your hand out, you could fall on your face. I think a broken wrist is better than head trauma.

There are two things I want you to remember about falling; protect your head AND protect your head. Landing on your hip is better than hitting your head. Technology can rebuild the hip but the head is another story.

There are balance training techniques that can reduce the risk of hitting your head if you lose your balance but those techniques are more advanced and require "hands on" training with a certified FallProof™ balance and mobility specialist who is trained to demonstrate and guide you through the processes.

In the meantime, practice your balance challenges, strengthen your body and stretch what you strengthen. Balance is a total body experience between mind and muscle so always protect your head.

## Medications That Increase Risk of Falling

Balance is an intricate messenger system that involves your mind, muscles and senses. The central nervous system regulates the speed and quality of information that is communicated through this messenger system.

The number one side effect of most medications is dizziness and if it doesn't make you dizzy, the medication will probably make you drowsy and slow down your reaction times.

Medications that affect your central nervous system increase the risk of an accidental fall.

If you're taking more than one medication that affects your central nervous system, your chance of falling is that much greater. Be aware of how each pill makes you feel and adjust your activity schedule accordingly.

Also be aware that drugs hang around longer in the older body because of declining liver and kidney function. Thus, the "adult dose" is half the recommended dosage. This includes over the counter medications. Talk to your doctor about appropriate dosages.

The following medications are known to increase fall risk:

- ACE Inhibitors (3)
- Alcohol (1, 5)
- Alpha Receptor Blockers (2, 3)
- Anticoagulants (8)
- Anticonvulsants (1, 2, 5, 6, 7)
- Antidepressants, especially tri-cyclic (1,2,3,6)
- Antihistamines, sedating (1)
- Cold Medications that contain sedating antihistamines (1)
- Antipsychotics (1, 3, 4)
- Corticosteroids, oral and inhaled, highdose (7)
- Digoxin (unknown effect)
- Eye drops (6)
- Herbal and Natural health products and sleep aids (unknown)
- Muscle Relaxants (1, 2)
- Nitrates (2,3)
- NSAIDs /ASA/acetylsalicylic acid, aspirin (8)
- Opiates/narcotics (1,2)

- Sedative/hypnotics, Benzodiazepines, Barbiturates (1, 2, 5)
- Thiazolidinediones  (7)

## POSSIBLE BODY MECHANISM CONTRIBUTING TO FALL RISK:

(1) Drowsiness

(2) Dizziness

(3) Hypotension

(4) Parkinsonian effects

(5) Ataxia/gait disturbance

(6) Vision disturbance

(7) Osteoporosis or reduced bone mineral density increases the fracture risk if a fall occurs

(8) Risk of serious bleeding if a fall occurs.

## Home Safety Checklist

<u>Stairs and Steps</u>

- Make sure light switches are at both the top and bottom of the stairs.
- Provide enough light to see each step and the top and bottom landings.
- Consider installing motion detector lights, which turn on automatically and light your stairway.
- Keep flashlights nearby in case of a power outage.
- Install handrails on both sides of the stairway and be sure to use them.
- If you have bare-wood steps, put nonslip treads on each step.
- Do not use patterned, dark, or thick carpeting. Solid colors show the edges of steps more clearly.
- Repair loose stairway carpeting or boards immediately.
- Do not place loose area rugs at the bottom or top of stairs.
- Do not leave objects on the stairs.

<u>Bathroom</u>

- Install grab bars on the bathroom walls near the toilet and along the bathtub or shower.
- Replace glass shower enclosures with non-shattering material.
- Place a slip-resistant rug next to the bathtub for safe exit and entry.
- Mount a liquid soap dispenser on the bathtub/shower wall.
- Place nonskid adhesive textured strips on the bathtub/shower floor.
- Use a sturdy, plastic seat in the bathtub if you are unsteady or if you cannot lower yourself to the floor of the tub.
- Stabilize yourself on the toilet by using either a raised seat or a special toilet seat with armrests.

<u>Bedroom</u>

- Clear clutter from the floor.
- Place a lamp and flashlight near your bed.

- Sleep on a bed that is easy to get into and out of.
- Install nightlights along the route between the bedroom and the bathroom.
- Keep a telephone near your bed.

## Living Areas

- Arrange furniture to create clear pathways between rooms.
- Remove low coffee tables, magazine racks, footrests, and plants from pathways in rooms.
- Install easy-access light switches at entrances to rooms. *Glow-in-the-dark switches* may be helpful.
- Secure loose area rugs with double-sided tape or slip-resistant backing. Recheck these rugs periodically.
- Keep electric, appliance, and telephone cords out of your pathways, but do not put cords under a rug.
- Place carpeting over concrete, ceramic, and marble floors to lessen the severity of injury if you fall.
- Repair loose wooden floorboards immediately.
- Throw away wobbly chairs, ladders, and tables.
- Do not sit in a chair or on a sofa that is so low it is difficult for you to stand up.

## Kitchen

- Remove throw rugs.
- Immediately clean up any liquid, grease, or food spilled on the floor.
- Store food, dishes, and cooking equipment at an easy-to-reach, waist-high level.
- Do not stand on chairs or boxes to reach upper cabinets.
- Use only a stepstool with an attached handrail so that you are supported.
- Repair loose flooring.
- Use nonskid floor wax.

## Senior Resource Directory

1.  **FallProof™ Balance and Mobility Program** (Dr. Debra Rose)
    - A multidimensional approach to the assessment and treatment of balance-related problems.
    - Developed at the Center for Successful Aging, California State University, Fullerton

    **Eligibility for community-based classes**:
    - Live in the community
    - Able to safely walk a distance of 200 feet without the use of any assistive device (cane or walker)
    - No memory loss or cognitive impairment likely to adversely impact judgment and/or decision-making abilities
    - No unstable medical condition (e.g., uncontrolled diabetes, cardiovascular disease, high blood pressure, or asthma)
    - Website: http://www.stopfalls.org

2.  **Matter of Balance** (Patti League)
    - Program designed to reduce the fear of falling and increase activity levels among older adults.
    - Website: http://www.mmc.org

3.  **Senior Fitness Tests** (Roberta Rikli and Jesse Jones)
    - A battery of seven (7) tests used to assess physical fitness in older adults, specifically the physical attributes needed to perform everyday activities
    - Chair Stand, Sit and Reach, 8' Up and Go, Arm Curl, Back Scratch Test, 2-Minute Step Test, 6-Minute Walk Test

4.  **Vision Specialists**
- Society for the Blind **(916) 452-8271,**www.societyfortheblind.org
- **Hearing Specialists**
    - Avalon Hearing Aid Center (family owned): (888-490-0056)
- **Footwear**
    - Dr. Basso's Midtown Comfort Shoes (916-731-4400)
    - Fleet Feet (916-442-3338)
    -

- **Medical Alert Systems**
  - Vital Link (800-752-5522)
  - Response Link (866-802-3676)
  - Lifeline (800-380-3111)
- **Medication Management**
  - California Poison Control (800-222-1222)
- **Home Modification Companies**
  - Rebuilding Together (http://rebuildingtogether.org/)
  - Home Safety Services (http://www.homesafety.net/)
- **Transition Movers**
  - Seniors in Transition (www.SeniorsInTransitionOnline.com)
  - Smooth Transitions-Sacramento (http://www.movingforseniors.com/)

## State and Federal agencies:

AARP (http://www.aarp.org)

California Department of Public Health (http://www.cdph.ca.gov)

Fall Prevention Center of Excellence (http://www.stopfalls.org)

Center for Successful Aging (http://hhd.fullerton.edu/csa/)

Senior Fitness Association (http://www.seniorfitness.net/)

## Support groups:

American Chronic Pain Association (www.theacpa.org)

Diabetes Association (http://www.diabetes.org)

Fibromalgia (http://rosevillefibromyalgia.com/)

Arthritis (http://www.arthritis.org/)

Neuropathy Association (http://www.neuropathy.org)

Crohn's Disease (http://www.ccfa.org/)

## Other sites of interest:

- **American Geriatrics Society Foundation for Health in Aging**
  http://www.healthinaging.org
- **American Academy of Audiology** (AAA)
  http://www.audiology.org
- **American Academy of Neurology** (AAN)
  http://www.aan.com
- **American Academy of Otolaryngology-Head and Neck Surgery**
  http://www.entnet.org
- **American Academy of Physical Medicine and Rehabilitation**
  http://www.aapmr.org
- **American Geriatrics Society** (AGS)
  http://www.americangeriatrics.org
- **American Otological Society and American Neurotology Society**
  http://www.americanotologicalsociety.org/
- **American Physical Therapy Association** (APTA)
  http://www.apta.org
- **Audiology Foundation of America**
  www.audfound.org
- **Gerontological Society of America** (GSA)
  http://www.geron.org/
- **Healthy Aging for Older Adults** (Centers for Disease Control)
  http://www.cdc.gov/aging/
- **International Council on Active Aging** (ICAA)
  http://www.icaa.cc
- **National Academy on an Aging Society**
  http://www.agingsociety.org/agingsociety/
- **National Institute on Aging**
  http://www.nia.nih.gov/
- **National Institutes of Health**
  http://www.nih.gov/

- **US Administration on Aging**
  http://www.aoa.dhhs.gov/
- **Vestibular Disorders Association** (VEDA)
  http://www.vestibular.org/
- **Administration on Aging**
  www.aoa.dhhs.gov
- **Alliance for Aging Research**
  www.agingresearch.org
- **Falls and Hip Fractures among Older Adults (National Center for Injury Prevention and Control)**
  www.cdc.gov/ncipc/factsheets/falls.htm
- **National Institute on Deafness and Other Communication Disorders - Health Information: Hearing and Balance**
  www.nidcd.nih.gov/health/pubs_hb/balance_disorders.htm
- **National Resource Center on Aging & Injury**
  www.safeaging.org
- **Senior Care Web**
  http://seniorcareweb.com/senior/mobility/default.htm
- **Vestibular Disorders Association (VEDA)**
  www.vestibular.org